Engineering and Living Systems

Engineering and Living Systems:
Interfaces and Opportunities

David D. Rutstein and Murray Eden

THE MIT PRESS
CAMBRIDGE, MASSACHUSETTS, AND LONDON, ENGLAND

R
856
.R87

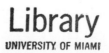

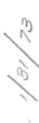

It is these boundary regions of science which offer the richest opportunities to the qualified investigator. They are at the same time the most refractory to the accepted techniques of mass attack and the division of labor. If the difficulty of a physiological problem is mathematical in essence, ten physiologists ignorant of mathematics will get precisely as far as one physiologist ignorant of mathematics, and no further. If a physiologist, who knows no mathematics, works together with a mathematician who knows no physiology, the one will be unable to state his problem in terms that the other can manipulate, and the second will be unable to put the answers in any form that the first can understand. . . . The mathematician need not have the skill to conduct a physiological experiment, but he must have the skill to understand one, to criticize one, and to suggest one. The physiologist need not be able to prove a certain mathematical theorem, but he must be able to grasp its physiological significance and to tell the mathematician for what he should look. We had dreamed for years of an institution of independent scientists, working together in one of these backwoods of science, not as subordinates of some great executive officer, but joined by the desire, indeed by the spiritual necessity, to understand the region as a whole, and to lend one another the strength of that understanding.

Norbert Weiner, *Cybernetics*, 2nd ed. (Cambridge, Mass.: The M.I.T. Press, 1962), pp. 2–3.

Acknowledgments

Acknowledgment is made to the many members of the faculties and administrations of Harvard University and the Massachusetts Institute of Technology, whose thoughts and ideas have influenced the form and content of this book. Particular appreciation is expressed to the members of the Joint Committee on Engineering and Living Systems for wisdom and guidance, to the Task Group chairmen and members for their careful formulation of the status of their representative fields, and to the Steering Committee and study staff for their enthusiastic participation in the creation of the original report ("Harvard University-Massachusetts Institute of Technology Program on Engineering and Living Systems" prepared for the National Academy of Engineering in Washington, D.C., September 30, 1968) upon which this book is based.

The authors are deeply grateful to Rita J. Nickerson for her statistical evaluations and to Ernestine Macedo for the typing of many drafts of this book.

We are grateful to the Committee on the Interplay of Engineering with Biology and Medicine of the National Academy of Engineering for the grant that made the original report possible.

Dr. Rutstein once again expresses his indebtedness to the Commonwealth Fund for the generous grant that provided administrative, editorial, and library assistance, secretarial support, and travel funds, lightening his administrative responsibilities and releasing his time for academic pursuits such as his share in the preparation of this book.

Cambridge, Massachusetts
April 1970

David D. Rutstein
Murray Eden

Contents

Engineering and Living Systems

Background

Our knowledge of living systems has been based, for the most part, on the tripod of anatomy, biochemistry, and physiology. The contributions of the physical and engineering sciences and mathematics have been relatively few, and their interrelationships with biology and medicine have been casual ones. It is the purpose of this book to indicate how the medicine and biology of the future can be built on a foundation consisting of all of these disciplines [1] in order better to understand the nature of health and disease in the individual and to design more viable and complete medical care programs.

This book is the authors' interpretation of the general principles that have emerged from the continuing evolution of the Harvard University–Massachusetts Institute of Technology Program on Engineering and Living Systems. The book is based on the Report to the National Academy of Engineering Committee on the Interplay of Engineering with Biology and Medicine entitled, *Harvard University–Massachusetts Institute of Technology Program in Engineering and Living Systems. A Joint Proposal for Education, Research, Development, and Medical Care to Interrelate the Physical and Engineering Sciences, Mathematics, Methods of Management, and Technology, with Biology and Medicine, September 30, 1968.* The authors were the co-principal investiga-

---

[1] It is recognized that the increasingly quantified and statistical approach to the social and behavioral sciences will yield benefits to human health and to the prevention and treatment of disease. However, a thorough evaluation of the contributions of social and behavioral sciences is beyond the scope of this book.

tors of that report. This text represents their personal views and is not an official document. With the permission of the chairmen, the sixteen original task group summaries in the report, which provide substantiating documentation, are reproduced here verbatim.

A Brief History

Both Harvard University and the Massachusetts Institute of Technology have made many contributions to public health and medical engineering. While the two institutions have progressed independently in response to changing social needs and their faculties' interests, their histories have been closely interwoven for more than fifty years. William Sedgwick, in 1912, organized a school of public health at the Massachusetts Institute of Technology. He was soon joined by Milton J. Rosenau, the first professor of preventive medicine and by George C. Whipple, Gordon McKay Professor of Sanitary Engineering, both of Harvard.

The School for Health Officers was for some years operated under the joint auspices of the Massachusetts Institute of Technology and Harvard University. This marked the beginning of the first formal training program in sanitary engineering in the United States. Subsequently, as the medical profession began to be concerned with teaching and research in public health, the Massachusetts Institute of Technology focused on milk and food technology and sanitary bacteriology, while Harvard, with its department of sanitary engineering (1911), its division of industrial hygiene (1918), and the new school of public health (1922) in the faculty of medicine, concentrated more and more on the sanitary

4

engineering and medical aspects of industrial and environmental public health.

A period of relative quiescence was followed by a spate of increased activity after World War II when both schools began to move into new areas of research and education that combine the physical and biological sciences. Each school took a series of formal steps, among which were: the introduction of biophysics at Harvard with the appointments of Arthur Solomon (1946) and Bert Vallee (1951); the establishment in 1952 of the Massachusetts General Hospital Physics Research Laboratory under the direction of Gordon Brownell, Associate Professor of Nuclear Engineering at M.I.T.; the creation in 1956 of the Eaton-Peabody Laboratory of Auditory Physiology at the Harvard-affiliated Massachusetts Eye and Ear Infirmary, operated jointly with the Research Laboratory of Electronics of the Massachusetts Institute of Technology; the inclusion of biomathematics into the Harvard Medical School curriculum by the Department of Preventive Medicine with participating M.I.T. faculty (1959); the creation in the same year of the Biomathematics Division of the Department of Medicine at the Peter Bent Brigham Hospital; the development within the Department of Biology at M.I.T. of a major emphasis on physical and molecular biology under the leadership of Francis O. Schmidt; and at Harvard, the unification of engineering activities in the Division of Engineering and Applied Physics which by its affiliation with the schools of medicine and public health provided the focus for the engineering aspects of biology and medicine.

A large number of collaborative and individual research projects emerged from the interests of faculty and students. These activities have served to strengthen the professional ties between the two schools. At Harvard, medically based studies have ranged from those of regional health care systems by Osler L. Peterson to the development of artificial internal organs and synthetic surgical implants by W. G. Austen at the Massachusetts General Hospital and William Bernhard at the Children's Hospital Medical Center.

At the Massachusetts Institute of Technology, investigations include: applied chemical engineering, such as Edward Merrill's studies of polymer and surface chemistry in biological systems; mechanical engineering, as represented by the investigations of Ascher Shapiro on heart assist devices and the hydrodynamics of peristaltic flow in the human ureter; and aeronautics and astronautics, as in the case of L. R. Young's research in modeling the vestibular system in man and its implication for the performance of pilots and astronauts in the control of complex vehicle systems.

At the Harvard Division of Engineering and Applied Physics, William Bossert, with William Schwartz of Tufts University, is developing new insights into kidney physiology; A. Pandicio is applying principles of instrumentation to biological investigation; and Norman Zachary is bringing the resources of the Computing Center to aid neurological investigations at the Massachusetts General Hospital.

In 1964, the Dean of Engineering, Gordon S. Brown, created the ad hoc Committee on Biomedical Engineering (later the M.I.T. Committee on Engineering and Living Systems) to conduct an inventory of research and course offerings and to determine the extent of faculty commitment and the potential for future growth of

6

biomedical engineering. A report, prepared by Dr. Philip A. Drinker, "Graduate Study at the Massachusetts Institute of Technology in Engineering and Living Systems," included a tabulation of existing research programs in biomedical engineering. As of 1968, more than 87 faculty and staff members—from eleven departments in the schools of engineering, management, and sciences and from six institute research centers—were actively involved in these studies.

Resources

The resources available at Harvard and the Massachusetts Institute of Technology for a collaborative program in biomedical engineering are unique in their variety and abundance. The principal medical resources within the Harvard community are encompassed by the Harvard Medical Faculties, including the Harvard Medical and Dental Schools and the Harvard School of Public Health, with their laboratories and teaching activities such as the newly formed Center for Community Health and Medical Care, the New England Regional Primate Research Center, and the teaching hospitals affiliated with Harvard: the Beth Israel Hospital, the Children's Hospital Medical Center, the Massachusetts Eye and Ear Infirmary, the Massachusetts General Hospital, the McLean Hospital, the Boston Hospital for Women, the Robert Breck Brigham Hospital, the Peter Bent Brigham Hospital, the Boston City Hospital, the Cambridge Hospital, the Massachusetts Mental Health Center, the New England Deaconess Hospital, the Mt. Auburn Hospital, and the West Roxbury Veterans Hospital. Resources at Harvard University in Cambridge include the Division of Engineering and Applied Physics, the Departments of

Biology, Biochemistry, and Economics, and the Kennedy School of Government.

At the Massachusetts Institute of Technology, there are: the School of Engineering, the Departments of Biology, Chemistry, and Nutrition and Food Science; academic research centers such as the Research Laboratory for Electronics, the Electronic Systems Laboratory, and the Engineering Projects Laboratory, which are interdisciplinary and include members from several academic departments; and the Sloan School of Management, which has resources that may well be instrumental in the modeling of health care systems and the development of better information processing and management techniques for the delivery of medical care. Research units affiliated with M.I.T. include the Research Reactor, the Lincoln Laboratory, the Instrumentation Laboratory, the National Magnet Laboratory, as well as many departmental laboratories not already involved in biomedical research but with resources of men and equipment that could contribute effectively in a joint program. Finally, the Joint Center for Urban Studies of Harvard-Massachusetts Institute of Technology, formed in 1959, has in recent years begun the design of regional and urban health information systems.

Collaboration with industrial groups has also grown. At Harvard, approximately half the 101 investigations reported in a survey of collaborative research (*Catalogue of Bioengineering Studies in Progress at Harvard Medical School*) prepared in 1968 by Dr. Joseph Parrish[2] involve substantial industrial participation. M.I.T., with its long history of cooperation with indus-

[2] Dr. Parrish was the Executive Secretary, Subcommittee on Research, Joint Committee of Harvard University and Massachusetts Institute of Technology on Engineering and Living Systems.

8

try, has a general liaison program with more than 100 large national corporations and a more specialized associates program with about 30 smaller companies, most of them located in the Boston area.

Implementation

In January of 1967, in order to explore ways in which the Massachusetts Institute of Technology and Harvard University could work together most effectively, Presidents Nathan M. Pusey of Harvard and Howard Johnson of M.I.T. formed the Joint Committee on Engineering and Living Systems (JCELS) under the joint chairmanship of Dr. Jerome Wiesner, Provost at M.I.T., and Dr. Robert H. Ebert, Dean of the Harvard Medical School (see Table 1). The charge to the committee stated: "Harvard University and the Massachusetts Institute of Technology have joined forces to explore the potential for the development of collaborative efforts looking to the establishment within areas of the two Institutions of long-range programs and short-term studies in education, research, and medical care."

The proposed exploration was implemented by the establishment of three ad hoc subcommittees in education, research, and medical care. The Education Subcommittee focused its efforts on the development of programs and curricula for educating different kinds of physicians and bioengineers. The Research Subcommittee was primarily concerned with identifying and characterizing the existing collaborative research efforts of the two institutions. The Medical Care Subcommittee concentrated on the evolution of a community medical care laboratory comprising the relevant disciplines from both schools.

Table 1: Joint Committee of Harvard University and the Massachusetts Institute of Technology on Engineering and Living Systems

Harvard		M.I.T.
Robert H. Ebert	Co-Chairmen	Jerome B. Wiesner
Elkan R. Blout		Robert A. Alberty
Harvey Brooks		Gordon S. Brown
M. Judah Folkman		Murray Eden
Alexander Leaf		Boris Magasanik
Henry C. Meadow		Walter A. Rosenblith
David R. Rutstein		Albert O. Seeler
		Irwin W. Sizer

Subcommittee on Education

Alexander Leaf	Co-Chairmen	Irwin W. Sizer
Bernard D. Davis		Murray Eden
Daniel H. Funkenstein		Boris Magasanik
Melvin J. Glimcher		Sanford A. Miller
Howard H. Hiatt		William M. Siebert
David D. Rutstein		Benson R. Snyder
		Jerrold R. Zacharies

Subcommittee on Medical Care

David D. Rutstein	Co-Chairmen	Albert O. Seeler
G. Octo Barnett		Murray Eden
Leona Baumgartner		Robert W. Mann
Myron B. Fiering		Erik L. Mollo-Christensen
John H. Knowles		Walter A. Rosenblith
Sidney S. Lee		Jack P. Ruina
Osler L. Peterson		Louis D. Smullin
Jerome Pollack		Benson R. Snyder
Mitchell Rabkin		Joseph Weizenbaum
Gerald Rosenthal		Leon S. White
Alonzo S. Yerby		

Subcommittee on Research

M. Judah Folkman	Co-Chairmen	Murray Eden
W. Gerald Austen		Robert A. Alberty
William Berenberg		Paul R. Gross
Elkan R. Blout		Edward W. Merrill
Myron B. Fiering		Ascher H. Shapiro
David D. Rutstein		John B. Stanbury

The conclusions reached by the Joint Committee on Engineering and Living Systems and its ad hoc subcommittees provided the groundwork for the contract study with the National Academy of Engineering.

In the spring of 1967, the National Academy of Engineering established the Committee on the Interplay of Engineering with Biology and Medicine to determine ways in which the national engineering capability could be directed effectively towards problems of health and medicine. The National Academy of Engineering contracted with the National Institutes of Health for the support of the committee. The committee agreed to consider such areas as the role of engineering concepts in advancing the understanding of biological systems, the use of engineering technology in the development of instruments and devices useful in biology and medicine, and the application of engineering theory and methodology to the development of medical care systems, such as hospitals and regional health programs.

In November of 1967, Dr. John Truxal, Chairman of the Committee on the Interplay of Engineering with Biology and Medicine, invited the presidents of the two institutions to submit a joint proposal for a study to determine how their respective universities might bring their resources to bear on the problems of engineering and living systems. The proposal was to include the determination of the most effective ways in which university activities in engineering and the physical, biological, medical, social, and management sciences could interact to attack urgent problems in medical and health care; identifying the available medical, industrial, and civic resources to assist the university in these efforts; and the definition of the administrative structure that would secure the most effective relationship among the institutions.

Professor Murray Eden for M.I.T. and David D. Rutstein for Harvard University, selected by the Joint Committee on Engineering and Living Systems as co-principal investigators, submitted a joint proposal to the National Academy of Engineering in December of 1967. They conducted a study in which the respective strengths and interests of the two institutions were identified and made recommendations as to how they might best be combined. The contract was awarded in March 1968, and the study proceeded according to the schedule outlined in Table 2.

With the approval of the Harvard-Massachusetts Institute of Technology Joint Committee on Engineering and Living Systems, a steering committee [3] was established. Initially, the steering committee, in consultation with the Joint Committee on Engineering and Living Systems, identified the major areas of interest. As information was compiled, it became clear that in view of the wide variety of interests of the faculties of the two schools, the steering committee could not by itself provide the authoritative grasp needed to make specific recommendations in the many fields. It became particularly difficult to assess future trends and needs. The study was therefore decentralized under the auspices of sixteen separate task groups, each representing one of the identified major areas of interest.

The chairmen of the task groups (Table 3) became the key interpreters of the Report. From the outset it was realized that because of the unique subject matter to be covered by each task group, its membership, organiza-

[3] The members of the steering committee included the co-principal investigators, Philip A. Drinker, Henry C. Meadow, Joseph F. O'Connor, and the study staff of H. Frederick Bowman, William H. Matthews, and David M. Ozonoff.

Table 2: Schedule of the National Academy of Engineering
Biomedical Engineering Study

March 1, 1968:	Award of NAE Contract to M.I.T.-Harvard, with Professors Murray Eden, Massachusetts Institute of Technology, and David D. Rutstein, Harvard Medical School, named as principal investigators.
March 1–May 15:	Formation of steering committee. Definition of fields of study. Selection of task group chairmen.
May 15:	Employment of administrative staff. Establishment of central office.
May 15–June 3:	Orientation of individual task group chairmen by principal investigators.
June 3:	Meeting of Joint Committee on Engineering and Living Systems and NAE task group chairmen.
June 3–August 1:	Task group meetings and preparation of reports.
July 22:	Site-visit by the NAE Committee and Gilbert Devey, Executive Secretary.
August 1:	Task group committee reports due.
August 1–9:	Steering committee review of task group reports.
August 9–23:	Compilation of first draft of report.
August 23–September 10:	Review of first draft by Joint Committee on Engineering and Living Systems.
Mid-September:	Meetings with interested industrial organizations to discuss areas of interaction and cooperation.
Mid-September–September 30:	Drafting of final report.
September 30:	Submission of final report to National Academy of Engineering.

tion, and schedule, as well as the form and preparation
of the reports, should be made the responsibility of each
Task Group chairman.

The task groups met over a period of several months
surveying their respective areas. The full task group
reports identify current intra- and inter-university research efforts, outlining important tasks in each field
and defining the criteria needed to establish priorities in
the order in which they might be undertaken. The task

Table 3: Task Group Chairmen and Their Areas of Study [*]

Edward W. Merrill	Artificial Internal Organs
Murray Eden	Bioengineering Curricula
Richard J. Wurtman	Biological Control Systems
Daniel D. Federman Paul E. Brown	Continuing Education
Stephen K. Burns	Diagnostic Instrumentation
William B. Kannel	Diagnostic Processes
Oleh J. Tretiak	Image Processing and Visualization Techniques
G. Octo Barnett	Medical Care Microsystems
Nelson Y. Kiang	Neurophysiology
Sanford A. Miller	Organ and Cell Culture and Storage
Alfred P. Morgan, Jr.	Physiological Monitoring
Laurence R. Young	Physiological Systems Analysis
John F. Rockart	Regionalization of Health Services (Macrosystems)
Robert W. Mann Donald E. Troxel	Sensory Aids
Melvin J. Glimcher Robert W. Mann	Skeletal Prostheses
D. Michael Young	Subcellular Engineering

[*] The membership of each task group precedes its report.

group reports were intended to serve as guides to the administrations of both institutions in the evolution of the program to which they are committed.

Discussions at the task group meetings among formerly isolated workers resulted in collaborative undertakings in several new areas. For example, members of the physiological monitoring task group are exploring the mechanism and management of respiratory failure. The task group on subcellular engineering has originated a study of a new system for the separation of molecular particles (molecular weights in the range of 10^5 to 10^8). The co-chairmen of the continuing education task group are designing programs of study for physicians at the Massachusetts Institute of Technology Center for Advanced Engineering Study. The National

Academy of Engineering Study also gave impetus to increased contacts with industrial concerns. A meeting [4] was held of representatives from industry and many of the members of the task groups.

The model program proposed in this book is a distillate of the bioengineering activities of Harvard University and the Massachusetts Institute of Technology and is documented by the individual reports of the sixteen task groups.

[4] See section on Development.

This book presents a model for the planning, implementation, conduct, and administration of major programs in engineering and living systems and will concentrate on general principles of widespread applicability. In any university, such general principles would be best implemented by taking advantage of local resources and by adapting to local needs; the Harvard University–Massachusetts Institute of Technology model is obviously not the only way in which such programs may evolve.

An effective university program in engineering and living systems demands the meticulous interweaving of two disparate groups of disciplines—biology and medicine on the one hand and the physical and the engineering sciences and mathematics on the other. These groups of disciplines have been related to each other ad hoc, and collaboration has depended mostly on informal personal relationships. At times, research combining these disciplines has been performed in specialty fields such as neurophysiology; development programs have yielded new medical machines such as heart-lung pumps; and a small number of strongly motivated graduate students have qualified in both fields by the long process of sequential matriculation in schools of engineering and medicine. However, the institutional structure necessary for an effective, broadly based, systematic collaboration in engineering and living systems has been almost entirely lacking.

At first sight, the addition of relevant medical school departments to a school of technology, or the creation of departments of physics, engineering, and mathematics within a medical school would seem to provide the necessary institutional structure. Upon closer examination, the requirements of such departments make their establishment and maturation for this special purpose a difficult task. Recruitment of faculty to narrow, specialized, and relatively isolated units would probably be difficult in competition with existing generalized departments in the same disciplines in schools of engineering or medicine. A procedure more likely to succeed would be to build a university program in engineering and living systems by bringing together relevant units of different schools within the same university—or as in this case those of different universities—and stimulating their interaction. The gaps in scientific coverage in the new program could then be filled in by the creation of new units. The Massachusetts Institute of Technology and Harvard University have been exploring this latter road to take advantage of their unique assets, to decrease duplication of effort, and to prevent waste of financial resources.

The choice of an institutional structure to implement the program presents a serious dilemma. Ideally, the institutional structure has one major objective—to achieve optimal benefits from the interrelated disciplines. Therefore, the institutional structure must have visibility, it must perform all necessary administrative functions, and it must supply financial support. But the creation of too strong an institutional structure, with its own intramural faculty, could inhibit interchange among competent and deserving faculty members who remain in other departments of the separate universities (or indeed in separate schools within the same university) and could deny them financial support. The stronger the intramural structure with separate administration, the more it resembles the isolated "Institute" in the European sense. Many questions are raised: Would not the professor of electrical engineering or physiology, for example, be cut off, in the intramural structure, from his own discipline as represented by the analagous department in one of the collaborating universities? Would not granting agencies prefer to allocate funds to the strong intramural unit rather than to individual investigators outside the center? Would not too rigid an institutional structure defeat the primary objective of attaining optimal exchange of ideas among the members of the two faculties?

A solution would therefore depend on the balanced development of an institutional form flexible enough to foster conditions favorable to a common intellectual environment and the interchange of faculty, disciplines, ideas, and resources, and yet strong enough to administer the program and procure funds. In any event, the institutional structure must serve the needs of the program. First, the program must be defined; only then can the institutional structures be designed to carry it out. The resolution of this dilemma will be the key to successful university programs in engineering and living systems.

Interfaces and Opportunities

The focal points for a university program in engineering and living systems are the interfaces between medicine and biology on the one side and the physical and engineering sciences and mathematics, with their technology, on the other. We have identified and defined five such interfaces: three are concerned with the immediate application of existing knowledge; one with the engineering approach to the solution of practical problems; and the fifth, with fundamental research.

At every interface, the electronic computer is an essential working tool. It has had a major impact on health science research and permits investigation of problems that could not be studied by manual methods. In the National Academy of Engineering study, no special task group was established on the use of the computer. Rather, each task group referred to the computer according to specific needs in its area of interest.

The Applied Interfaces

The first of the three interfaces, all of which are concerned with the application of existing knowledge, is the development of machines to be physically attached to the patient for the purpose of sustaining his life and health. Such a machine might be in the form of an artificial organ such as the kidney or heart, a feedback mechanism to control blood pressure or another human physiologic function, an electronic prosthesis to help paraplegic patients to walk, or a sensory aid to help the deaf to hear or the blind to read.

The second interface relates to instrumentation and automation and has two objectives in mind—to make precise and reliable measurements and to replace analytical functions currently performed by human beings. Improved analytic measurements may be attained by automation of such medical procedures as laboratory testing, covering the spectrum from the chemical assay of sugar in the blood and the counting of blood cells to computer-controlled scanning machinery for reading electrocardiograms and other records of physiological performance. Analytical instrumentation could aid the physician to make a diagnosis or a nurse to monitor a seriously ill patient in the hospital's intensive care or emergency unit.

At the third interface, management theory with the mathematical tools of systems analysis and operations research can facilitate the more efficient allocation of our limited medical and social resources in order to provide preventive and therapeutic care to the patient in a more orderly fashion.

Development is the fourth interface. Development is defined as the conscious search within the social and economic framework for practical applications of research knowledge in biology and medicine to improve human health and to prevent and treat disease.

The Basic Interface

The fifth interface, and the most important over the long range, concerns fundamental research to yield new knowledge in the physical and engineering sciences and to evolve new mathematical theory for the solution of biological and medical problems. Medicine and biology can be strengthened by supplementing the existing underpinnings of the anatomical, physiological and biochemical sciences with physics, engineering, and mathematics.

Theoretical Implications

Exchange of theoretical concepts across all of the five interfaces would enhance the opportunities for the interplay of engineering and the physical sciences with biology and medicine, both for research and for practical application. Each of the task group reports included in this volume reveals one or another such opportunity. Some of the specific proposals in the reports are ready for exploitation and could be carried out at the present time. Other special opportunities would be created if a common intellectual environment and a valid institutional structure are established to blend the appropriate amalgam of complementary resources, such as those of Harvard University and the Massachusetts Institute of Technology.

To illustrate, we may explore the parallel concepts of homeostasis in biology and feedback in engineering. Homeostasis implies that should a change occur in the internal milieu of an organism and if the organism is to survive, the disturbance of physical or chemical variables must be corrected, either to restore the former equilibrium or to establish a new stable state. When Professor Walter B. Cannon proposed homeostasis as the regulatory principle of physiology, he gave biologists both an important conceptual tool and a new insight into the control of function. In particular, homeostasis was useful as a principle that could replace teleological reasoning in the explanation of the interaction of functioning physiological subsystems, in much the same way that the concept of natural selection replaces the value judgments implicit in such statements as "the survival of the fittest."

Teleology is the word applied to the philosophical explanation for natural phenomena by regarding them as the consequences of a purpose or goal—that is, organisms are said to have developed pedal extremities for mobility, and plants develop chlorophyll for the use of carbon dioxide as a source of nutrition. Teleology was discarded as a mode of explanation in the physical sciences more than 200 years ago. Many biological phenomena can not as yet be explained in physical terms, with the result that teleological arguments are occasionally found in the biological literature of the present time.

However, with homeostasis as with natural selection, the concept by itself furnishes neither the scientific explanation nor the analytical instruments with which to seek an explanation. Merely applying the word "homeostasis" does not prescribe how the chemical and physiological interactions take place; nor does it provide the mathematical expression to describe the way in which equilibrium can be maintained. For example, a clinical investigator might observe that a patient suffering a specific loss of function, as might follow the removal of a particular endocrine organ, was still able to maintain life but at a different physiological equilibrium. The concept of homeostasis immediately suggests that control of the relevant physiological variables has now been taken over by a new mechanism. But the theory does not provide the information to decide whether the substitute controller is enzymatic, hormonal, neurological, or physical. Nor does it characterize the sensitivity of the new dynamic equilibrium in the patient to physiological or pathological stresses.

Cannon specifically, and correctly, ruled out thermodynamic equilibrium as the regulator of homeostatic balance, but he offered no other physical or mathematical explanation. Moreover, he did not seek out physical scientists or mathematicians for collaborative investigation into the exact mechanism of homeostasis.

There is a discrepancy in terminology that must be recognized if biologists and engineers are to communicate effectively with each other. A system that is in thermodynamic equilibrium is isolated from the rest of the physical universe; and such variables as pressure, temperature, and concentrations do not change with time. In contrast, biological systems during life are characterized by a continuous flow of mass and energy into and out of the system. When input and output are appropriately balanced, the biological system may be in dynamic equilibrium but will not be in thermodynamic equilibrium. Moreover, a biological system with input and output so regulated as to maintain constant values of such variables as pressure, temperature, and concentrations may be referred to in engineering parlance as a "stable system" even though it is thermodynamically unstable. Thus, the use of the term "equilibrium" by the biologist may be misunderstood by the engineer, and the engineer's reference to a system as "stable" may mislead the biologist.

During this same period, engineers were designing devices to keep the physical variables in machines from departing too drastically from the values adjudged to be optimal for performance. This concept has come to be known as *feedback*. Feedback is based on the principle that information as well as energy flow can be measured and that such information can be detected and used to control the flow of energy. Specifically, if a given level of energy expenditure (or chemical concentration, or speed, or any other dynamic variable) is to be maintained at a prescribed value, the feedback system must first measure the existing level, then compare it with the desired value, and finally use the difference or error signal to readjust the energy output to its appropriate level.

Curiously enough, the theoretical and mathematical principles underlying feedback were not studied explicitly by engineers until after homeostasis had been introduced into biology; this despite the fact that for more than 150 years feedback was the principle underlying the operation of motor governors and is essential to radio design. During the past 30 years, however, there has been an extensive exploration of the mathematics of feedback systems. As a consequence, explicit quantitative predictions of performance can now be given for a wide range of devices. The successful conduct of a space flight, for example, depends upon the accurate prediction and control of feedback of literally hundreds of specific dynamic functions for flight stability, accuracy of trajectory, maintenance of the capsule environment, and, indeed, the health and peace of mind of the astronauts.

Norbert Wiener, who made seminal contributions to control theory, was well aware of the relevance of feedback to biology. He proposed the word "cybernetics" to encompass the concepts that relate energy flow and information flow. His ideas formed the basis of a theory that enables man to control and predict the behavior of integrated systems of great complexity by correlating information on the environment and on inputs to the system with the knowledge available about the internal states of the system. He envisioned the development of a science of cybernetics that would not only be applicable to man's control of the tools of his own creation but would also provide for a deeper understanding of man himself.

Progress in the application of feedback to the life sciences has been very slow. Most feedback theory deals with linear systems, whereas biological regulation is almost invariably nonlinear.

The difference between linear and nonlinear systems can be demonstrated by the contrast between the behavior of an electronic circuit when current is introduced and the behavior of the blood glucose level of a patient following the ingestion of glucose. After the addition of an aliquot of current into an electronic device, the voltage output rises from zero to some maximum and slowly decays back to zero. After feeding an aliquot of glucose, the time course of the blood glucose level will have qualitatively similar behavior. If twice as much current is introduced into the circuit, the voltage output will have a value exactly twice that of the first experiment for every point along the time curve. In contrast, doubling the dose of glucose will raise the blood glucose time curve but not to twice the original level. Thus, the "dose response curve" of that biological system is nonlinear.

Furthermore, regulated variables such as chemical concentrations, pH, flow rates, and respiratory volumes cannot be quantified without the measuring device itself introducing substantial alterations in the biological system. Under the circumstances, it is not surprising that the biologist is likely to regard the engineer's interpolations into his affairs as simplistic. Conversely, the engineer suspects the biologist of deliberately interposing difficulties to avoid a revolutionary redefinition of his understanding of the problem. There may be an element of truth to both views. So far as control of function is concerned, confusion arises because homeostasis and feedback are not merely different restatements of the same idea. Rather they are complementary facets of a theory that has not yet been unified.[5]

Following upon the basic principle of homeostasis, observations of a particular biological function may establish the fact that a certain physiological variable has gone from one stable state to another. Feedback theory can now be applied to furnish the quantitative description of the control function and a description of its behavior under perturbation.

This example illustrates one area in which closely parallel theories have evolved in different disciplines with virtually no interaction. It illustrates further that collaboration between complementary disciplines such as engineering and biology could yield new theoretical concepts, in addition to solving practical problems. One may well wonder how the two concepts of feedback and homeostasis might have evolved had there been an institutional structure adequate to assure a freely permeable interface between biology and medicine on the one hand and the physical and engineering sciences and mathematics on the other.

[5] During the past few years, experts competent in both physiology and control theory have made much progress although a complete synthesis has not yet been achieved.

A Proposed Program—A Personal View

The objectives of a university program in engineering and living systems are the discovery of new scientific knowledge and the development of new technology and their effective application for human benefit. The program therefore must address itself to five areas of activity: education, research, development, information, and medical care. In a practical sense, the success of the entire program will depend upon the amount and quality of knowledge yielded by the research. Research will thus provide the foundation for the other aspects of the total program. In any scientific field, when the research begins to yield substantive knowledge, it becomes justifiable to evolve an education program and to design and teach relevant courses of study. To further the practical application of research knowledge, development must evolve to produce the necessary instruments. Information must be classified and disseminated to facilitate the integration of the many relevant disciplines within the university, and with industry, government, and the public. Medical care programs using technology, systems analysis, and operations research must be organized to apply medical knowledge in the most effective way. These five areas of activity are so interdependent that all must be encompassed within the program.

Education

The broad range of activity in a program in engineering and living systems demands an equally wide spectrum of professional personnel. In this educational program the personnel can be classified in three categories:

1. Full-Time Leaders in the University

Bioengineers—a group of experts, educated and qualified in different combinations of the specialties of physics, engineering, or mathematics on the one hand and biology on the other. The term bioengineer thus refers

We are restricting the term "bioengineer" to denote an expert with thorough grounding in specific aspects of both fields. An engineer may apply his same professional skills to problems arising from medicine, meteorology or city planning. A medical scientist can use electronic devices or computers to obtain data or analyze results with no knowledge of circuit theory or computation. We would not regard either as bioengineers. We prefer the definition of Weinman who stated: "Physiology and biomedical engineering cover at least by definition almost identical fields of interest." The bioengineer is ". . . one who approaches biological problems with the 'eye' of a physicist or an engineer, or looks at physical phenomena with the 'eye' of a biologist: in each case the starting point is the specific discipline." [6]

to a congeries of many specialists, such as chemical engineer-metabolic expert, electrical engineer-neurophysiologist, fluid dynamicist-cardiovascular physiologist, and systems engineer-medical administrator. Also included are those bioengineers educated in medicine

[6] I. Weinman, "From Medical Electronics to Biomedical Engineering," Proceedings of the 5th Convention of Electronic Control Engineering of Israel, Session 1 (Haifa, Israel, 1965), pp. 1–9.

rather than in biology who, as in the case of basic medical scientists, have elected not to practice medicine, such as the orthopedic surgeon-mechanical engineer, medical diagnostician-mathematician, radiologist-radiation physicist. The categorical title of bioengineer would apply to all.

Physicians whose premedical education has been in the physical or engineering sciences or mathematics, whose medical careers are built on the knowledge of both groups of disciplines, and who elect to practice academic medicine. This category, as in the case of the bioengineer, comprises specialists qualified in different combinations of specialties in both groups of disciplines, such as mechanical engineer-orthopedic surgeon, mathematician-medical diagnostician, and radiation physicist-radiologist.

2. Research Collaborators

Graduate physicians who plan to collaborate in research programs with physicists, engineers, or mathematicians and who need postgraduate education in the collateral fields;

Graduate engineers who plan to collaborate in research programs with physicians or biologists and who need postgraduate education in the collateral fields.

3. Practicing Physicians and Engineers

Practicing physicians, including specialists and generalists such as general practitioners, pediatricians and internists;

Practicing engineers who apply their skills to the effective design or production of new models, prototypes, instruments, measuring devices, or systems.

Recognition must also be given to the need for undergraduate and graduate education for practicing physicians who specialize in bioengineering and for practicing engineers who will devote themselves to the solution of hospital and medical problems—an area that sorely needs attention.

The number of professional personnel in all of these categories is insufficient either to take advantage of the many research and development opportunities of engineering and living systems or to put into full effect in medical care the many scientifically and socially worthwhile bioengineering proposals. Therefore, the educational program must be designed to meet both the quantitative and qualitative personnel deficits of bioengineering and should be implemented with all deliberate speed.

The newness of the field and the lack of precedent and experience rule out rigidly defined curricula, particularly in the education of the bioengineer per se and the physician whose premedical education is concentrated in the physical or engineering sciences or mathematics. A truly experimental approach is needed. In these educational experiments, the faculties will have to accept responsibility and create—one for each professional category—a series of parallel channels, each with its elective options. The faculties will also have to implement a mechanism for continued supervision and evaluation of both students and curricula.

Because the educational program is designed to meet the special needs of bioengineering, it does favor students who have made a clear-cut decision to enter this field. It is recognized that at matriculation a significant proportion of students will not yet have decided upon a definite career and that they will be unable to select a specific channel. For them, there must be available a neutral channel analogous to the classical undergraduate medical curriculum, supplemented by appropriate elective courses designed to permit the student to explore his interests in various career possibilities, including bioengineering.

Whenever in the course of his formal education the student does elect bioengineering, the system must be flexible enough to permit him to shift from the neutral channel to a definitive one, or indeed, from one definitive channel to another. It is not at all uncommon for a science student who is being educated as a physicist to switch over to a curriculum in engineering, or vice-versa. But this element of flexibility is a rarity in current medical education. Experiments in core and elective medical curricula do not substitute for clearly defined channels with elective courses leading to definitive careers. The proposed program will still require the student to make an unambiguous career choice at some juncture. Most important, students who have decided early on a direction for their careers will be given the opportunity to pursue their special goals, while the undecided are given an opportunity to explore.

The Bioengineer

The evolution of a successful program will depend on the emergence of leaders who can interrelate effectively the disciplines of the physical and engineering sciences, mathematics, and management, and also interrelate technology with biology and medicine. These leaders will form the keystone of the arch joining both groups of disciplines. Many of the pioneers in this field are now limited by their lack of educational background. The leaders of the future must be able to interpret findings in one discipline to representatives of each of the other disciplines; they must be able to "carry water on both shoulders."

For the education of the bioengineer, it is recommended that a Joint Biomedical Engineering Education Committee be appointed to represent both faculties, and that it have authority to select student candidates, make ad hoc decisions regarding curricular content, supervise a board of tutors, conduct examinations, and recommend to either faculty the granting of degrees. The meticulous selection of top-flight students is a sine qua non. Students may be admitted at any time during the course of their study, perhaps even in their first undergraduate year. The Joint Committee would also be responsible for continuous evaluation of the educational program.

It is likely that in the early undergraduate years the curriculum of the bioengineer will be fairly fixed by the need for basic courses in mathematics, physics, biology, chemistry, and the relevant field of engineering. But even here, it is unlikely that the basic courses in their present form will suffice, as they were not designed with the bioengineer in mind. The conventional basic courses will have to be redesigned in accordance with the principle that mathematics, physics, and engineering are to provide foundations for the biology and medicine of the future. The examples presented in the physical science classes should be relevant to biology and the life sciences. Moreover, the teacher of the hard sciences will have to become aware of the importance and complexity of biological variation and the use of quantitative information in probabilistic rather than deterministic models. This change in focus should not be difficult, particularly since theory in such fields as particle physics has been based on probabilistic models.

As the student progresses beyond his basic courses, his curriculum will have to be varied to meet his special interests. There cannot be one single curriculum because there is more than one kind of bioengineer. Moreover, the student will not, as in the past, complete his undergraduate engineering education before going on to medical school. Integration of course offerings from both schools throughout the entire curriculum becomes necessary. For example, if a student plans a career as an orthopedic surgeon-mechanical engineer, it may be desirable that in his third undergraduate year he take a course in functional skeletal anatomy at the medical school; at the same time the future electronic engineer-cardiovascular physiologist might be studying the physiology of the circulatory system. Those bioengineers educated in a specialty of biology may need no clinical training, while those seeking a career in medicine will require basic clinical education. Whatever the method of teaching, every student seeking a career in bioengineering should be educated to mastery of at least one engineering or scientific field and to comfortable familiarity with at least one life science, or vice-versa.

The style of teaching is also important. Several decades ago, engineering education shifted from a focus on facts and methods to the principles of physics, chemistry, and mathematics underlying its technology. Recently, medical education has been following the same trend. In both fields, many facts and a large dictionary of terminology must be assimilated by the student if he is to practice his profession effectively. Programmed teaching, in which the student interacts with the machine, could facilitate the learning of the new vocabularies outside the classroom. It remains for the teacher in the classroom to demonstrate how the facts become the sinews of the principles. With such an educational background, during the course of his professional life the engineer or physician should be able to adapt to the rapid and revolutionary changes in the practice of his profession.

A fundamental rapprochement is necessary if the bioengineer is to relate successfully to both fields. Many great recent advances in engineering depend upon mathematics and the quantitative knowledge in the physical sciences; concomitantly, revolutionary new concepts emerging from molecular biology have broadened our understanding of the life sciences. But these two patterns of thinking are not converging insofar as medical science is concerned. Students with basic education in the physical and engineering sciences report that medical school courses in biochemistry appear to be far removed from clinical phenomena and the practical care of the patient and that they are deficient as explanations for organ and system function. Conversely, students with backgrounds in molecular biology are satisfied that an ultimate understanding of normal and pathological states would be based on knowledge of molecular interactions. They see no need for altering their highly fruitful research paradigm by the introduction of what they consider to be overly simple physical or engineering concepts of complex biological phenomena.

The advancement of medicine may well depend on the synthesis of the biochemical and the physical points of view. Thus, the implications of hydrodynamic theory may be as important as the control of fat metabolism in determining the localization of an atherosclerotic plaque in a blood vessel, while the genetic variation of an enzyme system may change the physical characteristics of the circulating blood. Rapprochement demands a common language to favor a meeting of the minds of physical and biochemical scientists. Toward that end, curricular experiments in bioengineering are essential.

In this experimental teaching program, tutorial guidance is required. Tutors would be assigned; at least one from each relevant group of disciplines, selection to be based primarily on the specialties of particular interest to the student. The students, individually and in groups, would work with a tutorial subcommittee both for their own guidance and for evaluation of the teaching program. Such a system would also lend itself to student participation in collaborative research with an investigator in his own field of interest.

Finally, on the basis of the student's performance throughout his educational program, and following a successful oral examination conducted by the Joint Biomedical Engineering Education Committee, recommendations for granting the appropriate degree would be made to the faculty. After several years of experimentation, it should be possible to establish specific curricular policies to guide the education of the bioengineer.

Physicians with Backgrounds in Physical
or Engineering Sciences or Mathematics

Those students with backgrounds in the physical or engineering sciences or mathematics seeking careers in medicine will not become bioengineers. They will become physicians, and their curriculum must provide for a thorough clinical training. In that training, they must learn to interrelate their knowledge of physical and engineering sciences with the concepts of molecular biology to gain a more adequate explanation of clinical phenomena and to promote better care of the patient.

The constraints of the bioengineering curriculum also apply here. Lack of experience and precedents preclude a fixed curriculum for the physician whose basic interest is in the physical or engineering sciences or mathematics. As in the case of the bioengineer, responsibility would be delegated by both faculties to the Joint Biomedical Engineering Education Committee. The committee would select promising student candidates; make ad hoc decisions about curricular content; supervise a board of tutors; conduct examinations; recommend to either faculty the granting of an appropriate degree; and be responsible for program evaluation.

A beginning may be made by designing curricula that fit together existing courses in the life and social sciences with those already established in engineering, physics, management, and mathematics. Once again, current courses will need to be reexamined and modified to meet the special needs. Moreover, new courses, for example in physiologic control systems, will have to be devised. Interdigitation of courses in both schools would be the rule, but their selection and timing would be individually determined.

Eventually, a clearly defined course of instruction, in an integrated curriculum with elective choices, could be defined and fitted into the curricula in schools of engineering and medicine.

Physicians and Engineers who Contemplate Collaborative Research and Need Graduate Education in Collateral Fields

This rapidly growing category should present few difficulties. Both physicians and engineers will recognize their limitations, and each will want to learn enough about the other's field to conduct joint research on programs of mutual interest. It should be fairly easy to arrange the sequence of subjects required to qualify investigators to participate in collaborative research on questions that they have posed. The Joint Biomedical Engineering Education Committee could advise individual investigators on their educational needs. The faculties must assure enough flexibility in each student's program, and in the curriculum and its individual courses, to satisfy his needs and to grant credit to him.

Practicing Physicians and Engineers

In the education of the practicing physician, physical and engineering concepts relevant to the practice of general medicine and its specialties must be included in the curricula. In contrast, since there is no general practicing engineer, only those planning to specialize and practice in biology or medicine must have basic knowledge in those fields included in their curricula.

The regular curriculum of the physician in most medical schools lacks much of the physical, engineering, and mathematical knowledge that could be helpful to all physicians concerned with the practice of medicine. Similarly, most engineering curricula lack the biological and medical teaching that should lay the groundwork for the sound design of new biomedical models, prototypes, instruments, measuring devices, and systems.

If current practice in medical education were to be

followed, course contents of the disciplines of physics, mathematics, and engineering could be introduced only by adding still more elective courses. A curricular program that guides students along well-defined channels of study is much to be preferred because it would provide the flexibility necessary to accommodate new disciplines and new career goals. Engineering departments already provide parallel courses of study for their major specialties. Medical education has not yet evolved to the point of providing parallel channels of study to accommodate the widening spectrum of career opportunities now available to the graduate doctor of medicine. When such a system is developed, the curricula for students in every channel will incorporate the knowledge of the physical or engineering sciences and mathematics that is necessary for the effective practice of medicine in their fields.

There is an immediate need for physicians specializing in bioengineering and for engineers to be concerned with the solution of major hospital and medical problems. Their precise roles will have to be defined and an undergraduate and graduate educational program established. Eventually, to assure effective interprofessional collaboration at the working level, the undergraduate and the entire spectrum of postgraduate education will have to lead up to specialty board qualification for the physician and an equivalent mechanism for the recognition of the professional status of the engineer.

Postgraduate and continuing education for practicing physicians and engineers in the future must also include information from the collateral disciplines if members of each group are to remain abreast of relevant major advances in the other's field.

Research

General Principles

Traditionally, fundamental research in medicine has been grounded in the anatomical and physiological sciences. In recent decades, biochemistry has become the major premedical science and the focal discipline of biological research. The physical and engineering sciences and mathematics have been peripheral to the mainstream and have not been introduced systematically into medical or biological research even though a few investigators armed with these disciplines have attacked fundamental biological problems. X-ray crystallography and its mathematics have proved essential to the elucidation of the structure of protein molecules; the physical principles governing the movement of ions through charged membranes and statistical communication theory applied to the study of neuroelectric phenomena are providing new insights into the function of the central nervous system and the organs of special sense; and hydrodynamic theory has clarified our understanding of the circulation of the blood.

We are learning that mathematics is becoming increasingly helpful in many ways. Better hypotheses are being deduced to test by experiment biochemical reactions and enzyme functions, physiological phenomena, population patterns, and medical care systems. Multivariate analysis and sequential decision theory are aiding the biometrician in unraveling the complexity of biological interrelationships and often permit the laboratory investigator, the clinician, and the epidemiologist to study *in situ* a cell, an animal, a human being, or a population without resort to the creation of simplified, artificial systems.

All three disciplines together—physics, mathematics, and engineering—provide many of the tools for life and health scientists, including high energy sources of ionizing radiation (diagnostic and therapeutic), the ultracentrifuge, the electron microscope, the mass spectrometer, and the electronic computer. Nevertheless, these disciplines are yet to be applied to the life and health sciences in a concerted and orderly way.

The introduction of existing theories and methods from the physical sciences and engineering into basic biological and medical research is only the beginning. New knowledge of physics and engineering and new mathematical theory are needed for the solution of specific biological and medical problems. This is not a new concept—these disciplines have already been influenced by the life sciences just as the life sciences have been influenced by them. The evolution of mathematical statistics from Galton to Fisher was motivated by biological research; Volterra's studies on integral equations were stimulated by his interest in fluctuating animal populations; McCulloch and Pitts showed how neurons might perform logical functions and thereby touched off a considerable development in mathematical logic. Recent research in automata theory and formal languages was initiated at least as much by Chomsky's interest in understanding human speech and linguistic behavior as by the computer specialist's interest in creating a theory for automatic computation.

Thus, the program must allow for the inclusion of physical scientists and mathematicians who are attracted by the complex problems of living systems, who can seek novel physical explanations or construct mathematical formalisms in order to provide new insights into the solution of problems in biology and medicine.

Implementation

The administrative structure should provide facilities and resources to (a) increase the productivity of established investigators, (b) aid the formation of collaborative research teams for the exploration of new ideas, and (c) conserve expertise by establishing categories of appointment of four kinds of professional research workers: (1) faculty members in one of the existing departments of the parent institutions; (2) appointees of faculty caliber who do not fit easily into the departmental structure of either institution, e.g., a physician whose interests and principal competence relate to instrumentation for the analysis of biological components; (3) professionally competent individuals whose interest in education is limited to the guidance of graduate students and who wish to spend full time in academic research; and (4) full-time research workers with no interest in teaching, who conduct investigation at levels comparable to applied research and development programs in industry.

University biological and medical research is made up largely of individual projects, each being the invention of a faculty member, perhaps in association with a small number of his colleagues and graduate students. Such investigation ranges from theoretical to applied research, whether performed by individuals or in groups. Competent scientists working alone have had great success in fundamental research: Willard Gibbs working in complete isolation developed his concepts of thermodynamic statistical mechanics and the phase rule. On the other hand, there are basic problems that can be solved only through the interrelationship of complementary disciplines, by collaborating scientists working together with a common protocol of experiment. An example is the discovery of penicillin by Professors Fleming, Florey, and Chain. At the end of the spectrum in the applied area, there are narrowly focused experimental research and data-gathering projects that are goal directed. Individual therapeutic trials or collaborative drug testing programs such as the United Kingdom–United States Cooperative Rheumatic Fever Study are examples.

All these varieties of research patterns are necessary for the discovery of all of the kinds of new knowledge and new theory that must underlie a development program. Whatever the pattern, the principle that investigators in universities be free to work alone or in groups and to choose the subjects of their research must be kept inviolate. It is the responsibility of the administrative structure to facilitate compatibility among these different patterns of research in the same institution and to relate their harvest of new knowledge and theory to an efficient development program.

Development

Development has been defined as the conscious search within the social and economic framework for practical applications of research knowledge in biology and medicine. We distinguish between research and development although there is no sharp line dividing the two. In the proposed program, a close continuing interplay between research and development is crucial. For example, the development of a prosthetic limb with several degrees of freedom depends on research in the ways by which the amputee can control tension in his residual muscle tissue and substitute visual feedback (looking at limb position) for the normal kinesthetic feedback (intrinsic position sense). But there are distinctive differences between development and research. Development always has a specific goal and is not pursued for its own sake. Development can be justified only when the basic scientific knowledge already exists, when there is an explicit need for the proposed device or system, and when realization is economically feasible.

There is also a substantial difference in the organization for development as contrasted with research. Research may be conducted individually or collaboratively, but development programs need group planning, close collaboration, rigidly defined time schedules, and clear-cut apportionment of authority and responsibility.

There is little precedent for planned development in the biological and health sciences. By tradition, the biologist and the medical investigator discover new facts and integrate them into the body of existing knowledge and into the fabric of scientific theory. Medical investigators have not participated actively in development, that is, in the scientific, technological, industrial, and social process by which a theoretical concept becomes practically effective for all who might benefit from it. Indeed, the academic, governmental, and nonprofit organizations in which most such investigators conduct their research have not been adapted to, nor have they directly undertaken, substantial development programs.

The instruments and techniques of modern medicine have been invented mostly by physicians or engineers for whom development was only a part-time activity. Occasionally, an individual with a strong personal commitment who was affiliated with an academic, governmental, or non-profit organization, has succeeded in the practical development of special devices in his field of interest. Products have been developed in small laboratories in a few hospitals, universities, medical schools, and governmental research agencies. For example, the system of blood fractionation, yielding such products as human serum albumin and gamma globulin, was developed by Professor E. J. Cohn and collaborating members of the Department of Biochemistry of the Harvard Medical School. Such groups tend to be relatively small and severely limited to the kind and size of projects that they can undertake. Moreover, in clinical research, new devices and procedures tend to be introduced in piecemeal fashion. It is rare to find the engineering system approach applied to biological problems—an approach in which the steps in development are specifically ordered and in which there has been careful planning for the interaction of the various facets of existing and innovative technology.

There would appear to be a clear social need for

44

systematic rather than haphazard development in the health sciences in order to take advantage of the growing store of scientific knowledge. In so doing, a university setting is appropriate so long as internal arrangements and the tight scheduling of a development program can be made consistent with the freedom of members of the faculty to choose their own research directions and of the students to learn without being hampered by technical tasks.

Many projects can be identified that are likely to benefit from development programs relating engineering to the needs of medicine. These development projects depend in large measure on basic knowledge drawn from anatomy, physiology, biochemistry, pathology, and other preclinical sciences, and the technology of the classical engineering specialties.

There is one area of development that deserves special mention. We look forward to the conversion of biological knowledge into bioengineering technology, just as physical knowledge has been converted into engineering technology. Until now, biotechnology has been applied most extensively in the fermentation and food industries, waste disposal, the biological transformation of pollutants, and the production of antibiotics. The consummation of the marriage of medical scientists and biotechnologists should yield many human benefits and is long overdue.

Commercial enterprises have thus far contributed very little to the early stages of the development process. A small measure of "organized development" in biology and medicine has occurred in the pharmaceutical and hospital supply industries. Occasionally, a company for a small additional cost has adapted to medical use a device created for some other and often more profitable purpose. Thus, computer companies have adapted standard models to purposes as specific as the reading of the electrocardiogram. Yet even when a smoothly functioning medical instrument or system is evolved, tested, and validated, there may be no mechanism by which it can find its place in the practice of medicine.

American industry can provide for the need of the consumer if the device or system can be sold at a profit. But profitability per se cannot be the crucial criterion for the introduction of a useful device or system in medical care. Many specialized and valuable medical devices have very limited markets and are not likely to interest large manufacturers with the greatest competence and the most extensive facilities for medical instrument development, manufacturing, and marketing.

There have been many attempts in the past to interrelate universities and industries in the sequence of the planned steps from research through prototype development to full utilization of an instrument or device within the medical care system. However, we have found that many workers experience a profound sense of frustration and a conviction that much more could be accomplished if appropriate mechanisms for interaction were established. One need only look at the performance of such organizations as the Lincoln Laboratories or the Instrumentation Laboratory affiliated with the Massachusetts Institute of Technology to document the sharp contrast between planned development and the more casual approach now found in biology and medicine.

To explore the relationships in more detail and to identify potential gains and problems of university-industry interaction in biomedical engineering, a conference was held during the National Academy of Engineering study. Those invited included faculty members of Harvard University and the Massachusetts Institute of Technology, industrial collaborators in recent research projects, representatives of the Massachusetts Institute of Technology Industrial Liaison and Associates Programs, and other industrial officials. Some of the conclusions presented here emerged from the proceedings of that meeting (Appendix, page 295).

University-industry interaction in bioengineering is much less clearly defined than community-university interaction, especially with reference to medical care. Successful university-industry interaction will depend on better communication between university deans and faculty, practicing physicians, engineers, and industrial representatives; a precise understanding of the economics of research in and the invention, development, and manufacture of medical equipment; and the creation of an organizational structure in which academic and industrial communities can exchange ideas and interact effectively and profitably.

Collaboration in bioengineering among the universities, professions, and industry must begin with better communication. Each participant must become aware of the potential contributions of his collaborators and the constraints within which they must perform their activities. The traditional scientific freedom and relative isolation of the academic community, the ethical principles governing medical research, the requirement that engineering technology be built upon a solid scientific base, and the economic advantages and limitations within which industry operates must all become common knowledge. Such understanding will facilitate a clear-cut division of responsibility between academic and industrial collaborators during the planning period and throughout the course of university-industry development programs in bioengineering.

An information clearing house using a "yellow pages" system is a practical first step. Included would be the names, interests, and affiliations of individuals in the university, in medical care, and in the industrial sectors of the community. With such a resource, potential relationships could be explored, and collaboration could be facilitated at the very earliest stages of research and development.

As the government and the public become aware that collaboration between the university and industry in bioengineering development is desirable because it can contribute to the national good, they will need to face up to the economic facts. The process of transition from the initial conception of a medical device or system to public availability is long and expensive even if the research phase is financed independently. The costs of developing a prototype into a marketable instrument or evolving a management model into an effective medical care system are so large and the potential returns so small that industrial companies are unlikely to undertake them unless there is an adequate market for them. When a market was likely to be assured, as in the development of contact lenses, the project was undertaken by industry. In contrast, if an instrument were invented, for example, to type streptococci—essential only to several dozen professional epidemiologists in their research programs—it probably would not be developed by industry. In the latter case, the government would have to subsidize the cost of development and become the major consumer or, failing that, guarantee a minimum market. Thus, industrial participation may require that the government assume a role similar to the one they have played in military and in space development programs. To assure wise decisions in this complex undertaking, the governmental agency responsible for funding bioengineering research and development will have to recruit staff members qualified in mathematics and in the physical and engineering sciences.

The institutional structure relating medicine and engineering must extend beyond the university to provide the organizational base and the administrative supervision necessary for effective university-industry interaction. Under its supervision, the complementary resources of academic, medical care, and industrial institutions must be effectively integrated to gain the potential benefits of medical knowledge. Coordination of a wide range of many different kinds of scientific and technical competences is needed for success in bioengineering development.

Administrative supervision of the total development effort, including pilot plant operation, must assure a successful product to the ultimate user whether he be physician or patient. Supervision must span a wide range of activity. Included are the following: initiation of channels of communication between the essential operating units in a development program; establishment of liaison with those manufacturing concerns capable of producing a sufficient number of prototypes or of undertaking specific aspects of its development; assurance that knowledge yielded by research be made immediately available to prototype designers; alerting of research scientists to gaps in basic knowledge that could prevent completion of the development project; institution of licensing and marketing procedures to protect the equities of the innovator, the university, the industrial concern, and the public; contracting for such tasks as materials fabrication and prototype construction that can best be carried out by outside agencies, that is, by industrial concerns or by special laboratories such as the Lincoln Laboratory and the Instrumentation Laboratory affiliated with M.I.T.; conducting collaborative investigation with interested outside research groups competent in a relevant field; creating new research units within the institution to perform specific tasks; and the evaluation of prototypes for compliance with engineering specifications and for clinical efficacy.

The major administrative decision is the selection, from many possibilities, of the few development projects to be activated. Such decisions cannot be made lightly. Development is costly and time consuming, and it demands meticulous planning. The resources an institution risks in a development project is many orders of magnitude greater than the usual investment in a research project.[7] When the criteria of adequate basic knowledge, social need, and financial resources have been met and a decision made that a specific development project is to be undertaken, it may be many years and millions of dollars later before its success or failure can be determined with certainty. The administrative structure must have the flexibility to permit reassessments and new

[7] Total expenditures during the ten years of the United States Public Health Service Medical Systems Development Laboratory in the National Center for Health Services Research and Development study on Telephone Transmission and Computer Reading of Electrocardiograms have exceeded four-million dollars and do not include the large sums expended by the approximately one dozen industrial companies collaborating in the program.

scheduling decisions at each step along the way. Ultimately, a decision must be made that success is likely and the activity must be continued until the product becomes available, or that failure is probable and the investment must be written off and the project abandoned.

The successful synthesis of the more quantitative physical and engineering sciences and mathematics with the largely descriptive field of biology and medicine will require a free exchange of information among all participants in the program. That responsibility would be assigned to an information service operating under the aegis of the administrative structure. The store of information to be collected should include a historical summary of joint research accomplishments; the status of current collaborative research projects; potential resources in manpower and money for expansion of ongoing studies and the creation of new ones; the interests and competences of all potential collaborators in research, development, and industrial liaison (See yellow pages system, p. 48) and the state of planning and evolution of the total program. Information would be disseminated in three ways: upon individual inquiry; through an educational program; and by way of a consultation service. Many functions would be served.

Scientists seeking either to expand an existing study or to initiate a new one must frequently search for collaborators with differing but complementary basic competences and interests. The search may be both difficult and frustrating. A scientist will not always know how to look for the appropriate investigator in another discipline, particularly if he is seeking a collaborator in a field far from his own. For example, an engineer who believes he can apply techniques of wave-form analysis to the detection of cardiac arrhythmias will need to know how the specialty of cardiology is divided before he is likely to find an interested partner. Since the scientist engaged in such search has little knowledge of the complementary specialty, he is not equipped to evaluate the professional competence or special knowledge of the potential collaborator. Precise information from up-to-date resource files, supplemented by consultation by the staff of the information service should improve the probability of successful matchmaking among the different kinds of scientists needed to investigate a particular question.

But, how will the scientist learn that a particular discipline outside his usual cache of resources may aid him in his research? An educational program supported by a consultation service could make the health science worker aware of the potential contribution of a discipline previously unrelated to his research. Through periodicals and seminars, information could be disseminated about the design of collaborative research studies that have been successful in the solution of health related problems and also about analyses of the reasons for the failure of unsuccessful projects. An individual biological or medical investigator could learn how problems analogous to his own were clarified or solved by joint research with physicists, mathematicians, engineering technologists, and experts in the management sciences. In turn, and in the same way, representatives of the latter disciplines could be informed of the kinds of biological and medical investigations in which their knowledge and theory could be helpful. An educational program is essential, particularly during the formative stages, to a program on engineering and living systems, as an increasing number of faculty members become affiliated with it.

In addition to its matchmaking function, the consultation service, comprising representatives of the mathematical, statistical, and other relevant disciplines, could aid in the design of studies and the preparation of protocols of experiment. Consultation could thus augment the skills and knowledge of an individual collaborator, build mathematical models for better hypotheses to test by experiment, elicit ad hoc advice from consultants in disciplines not represented on the research team, and aid in the statistical analysis and processing of the data yielded by the study.

Finally, all interested parties should be able to keep abreast of plans and progress of the program. The information service could thus prevent false rumors, endemic to new programs in established institutions, that hinder individual program participation. A free exchange of precise information is essential to the accurate evaluation of manifold complex interrelationships that are the hallmark of a successful program in engineering and living systems.

Medical Care

Health Care and Contemporary Technology

To visualize the nature and scope of the problem of health care, it is essential to view the state of organization and technological development of efforts to satisfy man's basic needs in our contemporary society—food, clothing, shelter, and health. Recent (1968) personal consumption expenditures to meet these needs in the United States are found in Table 4.

The mechanisms for providing food and clothing may be grouped together. The systems satisfying these two human needs have profited more from our nation's technological and organizational development than have housing and health care. Many basic industries employ modern technology for the efficient production, processing, manufacture, and distribution of food and clothing. Housing and health care, on the other hand, are not so directly influenced by the mainstream of modern technological development. The basic technology of house construction has changed very little in centuries: a wider variety of materials is available, but organizational forms in the building industry have remained static. Attempts to change and improve the techniques of design

Table 4: Personal Consumption Expenditures United States 1968

Categories	Billions of Dollars
Food	115.0
Clothing	46.3
Residential construction [a]	28.8
Health care	38.6

[a] Expenditures are for residential construction rather than personal consumption.

Source: U.S. Department of Commerce, *Survey of Current Business* 49, no. 7 (1969).

and fabrication of structures in light of the needs of people and the potentials of modern technology have had only modest success. The health care "industry" is in a similar state. Indeed, it is even more difficult to find viable links between basic industrial technology and the current organizational concepts, styles, and forms of health care.

The importance of these comparisons lie not in perfecting the analogy but in helping to understand the difficulty, scope, and complexity of the problems. There are several assumptions, however, that we believe we can make.

The research upon which our present ability to treat disease and maintain health is based stems largely from two sources. On the one hand, our ability to treat disease emerges from the work of biologists, medical scientists, and physicians in academic, governmental, and other nonprofit institutions. This work is directed almost entirely toward an improved understanding of what underlies life processes and of the life processes themselves in normal and disease states. The major disciplines are anatomy, physiology, and biochemistry, including molecular biology. On the other hand, the sanitary engineer and the epidemiologist conduct research in preventive medicine, that is, the conditions under which health is protected and disease transmitted. As with research in curative medicine, research in preventive medicine has usually been performed under the auspices of a governmental agency or a nonprofit institution.

With improved understanding has come greater ability to treat and prevent certain types of disease. But with the exception of minor activities in the pharmaceutical industry, very little research bearing directly on health

56

and health care is carried on outside the academic or governmental nonprofit framework. Furthermore, the practice of preventive medicine and public health is conducted almost entirely by national and international governmental agencies and private foundations.

The institutions in the United States that form the present principal basis of medical care, in contrast with prevention, are our community hospitals—large, small, teaching, private, municipal, state, and federal. From the point of view of their philosophy, organization, and relationship to society, they are the almost unevolved lineal descendants of their ancestors of the sixteenth century. Preventive services in hospitals have been virtually neglected. Indeed, the current status of curative medicine as the main foundation of health care systems needs to be reexamined and revised. Curative medicine is especially valuable in acute reversible disease, such as, infection, while chronic illnesses such as coronary disease and invasive cancer must be prevented. This concept is not fanciful. For example, the risk of coronary disease can be decreased and that of lung cancer almost entirely eliminated by not smoking cigarettes. As time goes on, the control of the latter group of diseases will continue to increase in importance. Health maintenance, disease prevention, and environmental control in developed or developing countries must begin to take their proper places in the health care structure.

The need for a reorientation in our institutional structures and in the nature of their services is evident, but the available resources are by no means unlimited. In planning the evolution of institutional and organizational forms, it is essential to select those techniques and methods that assure the best utilization of resources, particularly human ones, and the most effective and economical delivery of total health care. Equally important is the integration of these institutional, organizational components and resources into a health care system flexible enough to take advantage of new knowledge and new technology.

Leadership in health care must be vested in those whose education, interests, and experience equip them to deal with the total problem. The education, point of view, knowledge, and experience of the engineer, the management expert, and the physician must be integrated to assure leadership in this field. To generate such individuals is an important educational task for the universities.

Medical Care Systems

The approach to be outlined here is applicable to prototypes of a complete medical care system as well as to those of its subunits, that is ambulatory health care clinics, emergency systems, satellite and neighborhood clinics, nursing stations, specialty laboratories and medical information storage and routing systems. The operation of such a system will require a constellation of many kinds of personnel whose activities will have to be correlated for the care of each patient by his physician.

Medical schools have been assuming an ever-widening role in guiding the evolution of medical care from a cottage industry to an orderly system that uses to advantage modern science, technology, and management practice. The schools are beginning to recognize that research in medical care is essential if the patient is to receive the benefits of modern medicine. In this research, the mechanisms by which medical care is provided will have to be studied as precisely as we now investigate the mechanisms of diseases we wish to prevent or treat. We must have reliable information upon which to plan and proceed.

A program in engineering and living systems has a crucial role to play in the improvement of medical care. The physical and engineering sciences and mathematics can yield theory, tools, products, and logistic concepts to aid in providing medical care more equitably and economically. Technology by itself can now be used by engineer-physicians to automate preventive, diagnostic, and therapeutic procedures. It can also supply instruments to help alleviate the critical shortage of medical and paramedical practitioners.

A body of knowledge directly applicable to medical care is evolving through the development of models as employed in operations research or systems analysis as adjuncts to management theory. This approach is particularly useful when the resources to meet a complex need are limited. Operations research was born out of the military crises in World War II, in the hope that mathematical analysis of logistic problems would result in more effective deployment of the limited numbers of troops and stores of materiel. The military successes led to the application of these techniques to managerial problems in industrial production, business, and economic planning. Now they are beginning to be applied to public health and medical care.

Medical care problems are similar to the military ones in that two kinds of major questions have to be answered. They are:

1. How does one assess the relative costs and returns of alternative programs that must draw upon limited

resources in funds, material, and trained manpower?

2. How shall available resources be allocated and applied once a decision on priorities has been made?

Although the management disciplines in the area of medical care are as yet unproven, they should contribute to a more effective deployment of existing scientific, medical, and social resources in programs for the maintenance of health, the prevention and treatment of disease and disability, and the postponement of untimely death. Experimentation is essential.

As in the military situation, two kinds of information are required to construct a model: a precise definition of the medical need and an inventory of medical and social resources. Such information has to be collected and analyzed through studies carried out by specialists in epidemiology, sociology, biostatistics, and medical practice. To assure the relevance of the data, model builders should participate in the design of the studies. Medical care standards will have to be defined in order to evaluate the data and the validity of the models and also to serve as a scale for measuring the quality of medical care provided to the individual patient.

As an example, in the Harvard University-Massachusetts Institute of Technology complex, data collection and analysis might be performed by such units as the Center for Community Health and Medical Care, while the models could be formulated in the Sloan School of Management at Massachusetts Institute of Technology and the Harvard Division of Engineering and Applied Physics. To establish relevant standards, a clinical advisory committee could be selected from the medical faculty for clinical aspects and from engineering and management faculties for systems of quality control. Designing and planning such a medical care program would provide an excellent opportunity for substantive university-hospital-community interaction. Representatives of the community at large and officials of the hospitals and other medical care institutions would participate in every aspect of the planning.

PRECISE DEFINITION OF THE MEDICAL PROBLEM

In outlining the steps to be followed, we have chosen a specific example. Let us consider how data collection and model building might proceed if the goal were to plan and implement the Regional Care Program Legislation (Public Law 89–239). That legislation was designed to bring to residents of the United States, wherever located, the benefits of modern medical science to prevent and treat chronic illnesses, particularly heart disease, cancer, and stroke. It is not possible in a single study to obtain a sufficiently precise estimate of the community need for medical care. Instead, it is necessary to perform a set of studies to zero in on a fairly precise estimate of need. These studies include:

1. THE BURDEN [8] OF FATAL ILLNESS AND THE NUMBER OF LIVES THAT COULD BE SALVAGED

The burden of fatal illness can be measured by the design used so successfully in maternal and infant mortality studies.[9] In those studies, a group of specialists made immediate and thorough clinical investigations of all deaths in a defined region. Preventable deaths were

[8] As used in this work, the term "burden" refers to the consequences to the community imposed by unnecessary illness and death.

[9] New York Academy of Medicine Committee on Public Health Relations, *Maternal Mortality in New York City. A Study of All Puerperal Deaths 1930–1932* (New York: The Commonwealth Fund, 1933).

identified, their causes isolated and eliminated. As a result maternal and infant mortality rates sharply decreased.

In the case of the Regional Medical Program, each death in the categories of heart disease, cancer, and stroke would be identified from death certificates and subjected to immediate intensive, on-the-spot investigation by a team consisting of all the relevant specialists to ascertain whether the patient had indeed died of heart disease, cancer, or stroke (and if so, specify the exact diagnosis) and if all of the resources of modern medicine had been made available to him. If the number of deaths is too large for an intensive study of every death, the investigation is made on a random sample large enough to ensure statistical validity.[10] With such data, the total and preventable burden on the community of fatal illness in each category can be determined. An estimate can then be made of the proportion of persons whose lives might have been saved had they received optimum medical care as defined by the study.

2. THE BURDEN OF SERIOUS NONFATAL ILLNESS

An estimate of the burden of serious nonfatal illness in a particular community can also be made, as demonstrated by the studies of the Manchester-Uppsala-Har-

---

[10] The sample of deaths for investigation must be carefully selected. In the case of heart disease, cancer, and stroke, valid estimates of both the burden of fatal illness and the number of lives salvaged may be derived from a thorough investigation of a random sample of the death certificates specifying a cause of death under the rubrics designating these diseases in the International List of the Causes of Death, plus a random sample of all other death certificates to identify the false negatives, that is, those deaths from heart disease, cancer, or stroke in which such causes of death were not so specified by the physician on the death certificate.

vard Research Group.[11] A study of hospital discharge
records in all of the hospitals to which cases from the
region are referred should provide valid estimates in
specific categories of the burden and nature of serious
and nonfatal illness in the area served by the regional
program.

3. THE TOTAL BURDEN OF FATAL, SERIOUS, AND MINOR ILLNESS

The combined estimates of fatal and serious nonfatal
illness are adequate for planning a medical care program for most diseases. However, an estimate of minor
illness may be essential for certain widespread and
usually nonfatal diseases, for example, the common
cold, or for illnesses whose major manifestation is severe disability, such as arthritis.

Estimates of minor illness are difficult to obtain. In
contrast to the studies of fatal and serious nonfatal disease, estimates of minor illness require a population
survey, with its attendant high cost and the awkwardness
of interviewing many residents. When estimates of
minor illness are necessary, the studies might well be
performed in collaboration with the National Center for
Health Statistics, since this agency of the Department of
Health, Education, and Welfare has developed methods
and maintains mobile facilities for sample area-wide
surveys.

4. THE FLOW PATTERNS OF MEDICAL CARE

The first three studies count the number of people who
are ill and in need of care. Estimates must also be made
of the ways in which community resources are used for

[11] R. J. C. Pearson, B. Smedby, R. Berfenstam, R. L. F. Logan, A. M.
Burgess, Jr., and O. L. Peterson, "Hospital Caseloads in Liverpool, New
England and Uppsala: An International Comparison" (Lancet 2: 1968),
pp. 559–566.

medical care. Such estimates are especially needed in metropolitan areas, where patients are referred to any of a wide variety of medical care resources.

Patient-origin studies of representative samples of individuals referred to and from medical institutions or physicians should provide information about the pathways that patients now travel to receive specific services. Such studies cannot be limited to individual communities, because flow patterns frequently override geographical boundaries. For example, residents of Cambridge are often referred to teaching hospitals, to specialized institutions such as the Massachusetts Eye and Ear Infirmary, and to individual specialists in the Boston metropolitan area.

Data collected in flow-pattern studies can provide estimates of the proportionate burden of a particular health problem carried by a specific institution. Such data will be valuable in relating needs to resources and in planning optimal patterns of referral.

5. THE TOTAL ECONOMIC BURDEN OF ILLNESS

In addition to measuring the burden of disease per se, it is necessary to estimate the economic burden of illness. Methods are being developed to measure the total economic burden of illness in hospitals.[12] It is likely that the same methods will be applicable to estimate the total economic impact of specified illness in an entire region.

6. ADDITIONAL COSTS IN MONEY AND PERSONNEL OF SUPERSPECIALISTS' SERVICES

Modern medicine has fostered the development of a number of costly and complex specific kinds of treatment. The inefficient use of such services in our hospitals

[12] Personal communication from G. Rosenthal, A. M. Burgess, Jr., J. Carr, and O. L. Peterson.

is illustrated by their unrestricted proliferation—radiation therapy for example—in many of our metropolitan areas. This is in sharp contrast with the practice in Sweden, where superspecialists' facilities are created and located in accordance with the expected case load. Methods have been developed here for estimating the costs of establishing and operating some services such as renal dialysis [13] and open-heart surgical units and relating them to potential patient loads. Such cost analyses remain to be done, and data so collected should be most useful in providing a more orderly distribution of superspecialists' facilities in the United States.

These six studies are representative of the kinds of bracketing investigations that can delineate the nature of the medical problem in a specified geographic area.

INVENTORY OF MEDICAL RESOURCES

The following set of studies should provide estimates for an inventory of medical care resources to be related to the data collected regarding medical care needs.

1. HOSPITAL AND OTHER INSTITUTIONAL RESOURCES

As medical care becomes more complex and specialized, medical institutions become more varied in their structure and function. Very few hospitals, for example, are now prepared to provide all of the kinds of care needed to prevent and treat all diseases and maintain the health of all people of the community served by the hospital. It is difficult to describe exactly which services a particular hospital or institution is prepared to provide. Nevertheless, a beginning has been made in the previously mentioned tri-country (Sweden, United Kingdom, and

[13] Carl W. Gottschalk, chairman, *Report of Committee on Chronic Kidney Disease*, submitted to the Bureau of the Budget, September 1967.

United States) study to develop methods for quantitative and qualitative evaluation of the availability and effectiveness of institutional resources.[14]

It is clear that estimates of available resources alone will not suffice. Instead, evaluation must also include estimates of the amount and kinds of services made available through the resources in the existing institutions. Institutional resources have to be evaluated in terms of average and peak load. When services are inadequate, assessments of needed additional resources and their costs will have to be made. Much remains to be done before institutional inventory data will have satisfied the needs of the model builders.

2. PERSONNEL RESOURCES

Interest in the efficient use of medical and paramedical personnel has been stimulated by the report of the National Advisory Commission on health manpower.[15] Personnel studies often relate to a population base specific categories of physicians and other health manpower, for example, the doctor:population ratio. Whereas such ratios have been shown to be poor indices of the quality of medical care,[16] they do yield interesting and pertinent facts, for example, the tri-country study's disclosure that there are more qualified surgeons in New England,[17] with a population of eight million, than in England, which has a population of fifty million. This fact points up the need for clarifying studies to determine the rela-

[14] Pearson, et al., "Hospital Case Loads."

[15] National Advisory Commission on Health Manpower. *Report* (Washington, D.C., 1967).

[16] David D. Rutstein, *The Coming Revolution in Medicine* (Cambridge, Mass.: The M.I.T. Press, 1967), pp. 57–62.

[17] These figures exclude Connecticut, which in the regional medical program is included in the New York medical marketing area.

tive rates of operative intervention in particular diseases and of deaths from surgical illnesses, the relation between the patient's economic status and the frequency of surgical operations, and the possibilities of eliminating unnecessary surgery.

Studies of medical and paramedical personnel should include, but cannot be limited to, the effective use of each category of personnel. Many tasks now being performed by physicians and nurses in civilian medical care do not demand their professional competence and are wasteful of their time. It is reasonable to assume that such tasks could be taken over by others with less education and experience. Indeed, the National Academy of Sciences, in collaboration with the Surgeons-General of the three armed services, has initiated an inquiry to determine whether certain tasks now performed by physicians in the civilian population can be performed by nonphysicians as they are now being performed by medical corpsmen in the armed services.

Additional studies should be made to determine how well such tasks are performed in the military services and whether or not it would be possible to have them performed in the civilian population by specially trained personnel working under medical direction. Such reallocation of tasks should increase the coverage capable of being provided by the pool of practicing physicians in the country. Indeed, practical operating examples already exist. In the M.I.T. Health Service, nurses have replaced physicians in the performance of a carefully selected set of diagnostic and therapeutic tasks and continue to perform this function effectively under the direction of the institute physicians.[18]

[18] Personal communication from A. Seeler.

Resource studies will have to identify the quality and quantity of personnel in each professional and vocational category, both in and out of the hospital. The data collectors and model builders will need to work closely with clinical collaborators to determine whether the number of personnel in each category is adequate to meet the requirements for good medical care; the tasks performed by each category of personnel are appropriate to their education and training; new categories of personnel should be created, either by splitting up old ones [19] (nursing now ranges all the way from practical nurse to coronary unit supervisor) or by the creation of new ones (e.g., computer programmer or heart-pump technician); and tasks that do not require the education and training of personnel in one professional category can be transferred to less extensively educated and trained personnel, including technicians, or to machines.

Data collected in studies performed in local areas can be the basis for a more precise classification of medical and other health personnel. In each category, the task performed can be made congruent with educational requirements and salary levels.

3. TOTAL FINANCIAL RESOURCES

To round out the inventory studies, information is needed on the financial resources immediately or potentially available for preventive and therapeutic medical services in a particular region. Methods for the collection of such data have been outlined.[20]

[19] David D. Rutstein, *The Coming Revolution in Medicine.*
[20] H. E. Klarman, J. O.'S. Francis, and G. D. Rosenthal, "Cost Effectiveness Analysis Applied to the Treatment of Chronic Renal Disease" *Medical Care* 6 (1968) : 48–54.

One currently important program has been discussed in detail to illustrate a set of studies that are fundamental to the development of a model of a medical care system. This set of studies demonstrates that collaboration between groups of disciplines in a program of engineering and living systems may provide the key to an otherwise intractable problem. We believe the approach outlined here is applicable to prototypes of a complete medical care system as well as to those of its subunits, that is, ambulatory health care clinics, emergency wards, satellite and neighborhood clinics, nursing stations, specialty laboratories, and medical information, storage and routing systems. If new and successful medical care programs are to be developed, a close working relationship must evolve between the data collectors and the model builders. Thus, in the very design of the study the model builders would indicate the kinds of data that would be most useful for them. On the other hand, as data are collected the model builders can test and refine their models, describe the provisional consequences of the model's performance, and perhaps ask for additional or more precise or relevant data.

Throughout the evolution of a model medical care system, that model should be exposed to the scrutiny of a competent medical advisory committee to determine if it is, in fact, relevant to the practical management of the individual patient. When the model or specific parts of it are satisfactory to both the model builders and the data collectors and meet this final clinical criterion, they may be simulated on a computer or field tested in a community. For the latter purpose, it is evident that representatives of the local medical profession and of the community must be brought into the model building process at a very early stage.

This plan for the establishment of a medical care system makes it clear that work of direct relevance to the betterment of health can be a major ingredient of a program in engineering and living systems.

Summary

The total program of engineering and living systems is a university responsibility, to be coordinated with appropriate community agencies and industrial organizations and supervised by an institutional structure flexible enough to create a common intellectual environment and favor an optimal interplay of faculty, disciplines, ideas, and resources, but strong enough to provide leadership, administer the program, and guarantee financial support. As in the case of the Report to the National Academy of Engineering on the *Harvard-M.I.T. Program in Engineering and Living Systems,* this comprehensive conclusion requires documentation by representatives from the many disciplines involved in a university program on engineering and living systems. There follows the individual task group reports from the Harvard–M.I.T. Report, to provide such documentation.

Task Group Reports

Artificial Internal Organs
Bioengineering Curricula
Biological Control Systems
Continuing Education
Diagnostic Instrumentation
Diagnostic Processes
Image Processing and Visualization Techniques
Medical Care Microsystems
Neurophysiology
Organ and Cell Culture and Storage
Physiological Monitoring
Physiological Systems Analysis
Regionalization of Health Services (Macrosystems)
Sensory Aids
Skeletal Prostheses
Subcellular Engineering

Task Group Report on Artificial Internal Organs

Edward W. Merrill
PROFESSOR OF CHEMICAL ENGINEERING
MASSACHUSETTS INSTITUTE OF TECHNOLOGY, CHAIRMAN

W. Gerald Austen
PROFESSOR OF SURGERY
MASSACHUSETTS GENERAL HOSPITAL

Judah M. Folkman
ASSISTANT SURGEON
BOSTON CITY HOSPITAL

John P. Merrill
ASSOCIATE PROFESSOR OF MEDICINE
PETER BENT BRIGHAM HOSPITAL

Edwin W. Salzman
CLINICAL ASSOCIATE IN SURGERY
BETH ISRAEL HOSPITAL

The ideas expressed below are addressed particularly to the following paragraphs on page six of the communication from Dr. John G. Truxal to President Howard W. Johnson.

"Subcontract studies are expected to produce the following:

1. Prototype concepts for functional, organizational, and operational relationships of university activities in engineering and in the physical, biological, medical, social, and management sciences. Plans are to be directed toward securing the most effective interplay of these fields in the advancement of medical and biological research, in the development of practical solutions to urgent problems in the medical and health care areas, and in the enhancement of training of scientists, engineers, technicians, and instructors, who will advance multidisciplinary programs.

2. Identification and assessment of particular industrial and civic resources in the locale of the university that can contribute to exploiting the interplay of engineering, biology, and medicine. . . . Definition of problems which are amenable to solution via multidisciplinary efforts involving medicine and engineering."

1. Definition of Artificial Organs

In respect to this draft, sensory aids (e.g., artificial ears) are excluded because they fall into a separate category being worked on by another task group. Internal organs with very complex biochemical functions, such as the liver and the spleen, are arbitrarily omitted because at this time much more basic research is needed before a program can be intelligently launched.

Organs to be considered are those whose chemical functions are relatively simple, such as the heart, lung, and kidney (glomerular part only). Assuming these to be of immediate interest because of proven feasibility or near-feasibility, one perceives that they have in common their function in contact with blood under *in vivo* circulation conditions; therefore, biomaterials are significantly, though by no means exclusively, involved in their development.

Presumably, before any multidisciplinary organization can be brought to bear on the development of an artificial internal organ, a person or a group must evolve precise ideas of the design of the organ, so one can decide what services, such as industrial art, technician specialty, and so on, are required. Assume, for example, that a dialysis membrane will be used in an artificial kidney. If the membrane is in the form of flat cellophane sheets, as in wide commercial manufacture, the problem of assembling these sheets into various configurations is already almost eliminated. If, on the other hand, the concept calls for producing membranes of hollow fibers (Dow-type kidney), one must then be prepared to manufacture by extrusion, or some other process, the polymeric substance in the correct shape, size, and quality. Or, if the concept calls for a totally new configuration —for example, a helically wound tube—then a different and new manufacturing procedure will have to be invoked, requiring quite different fabrication techniques. In brief, *it would be wasteful to mount a large-scale effort until a basic concept has been carefully evolved and subjected to critical conceptual evaluation.*

By conceptual evaluation, we mean a theoretical analysis of how the device ought to perform if built (to get order of magnitude quantities such as square meters of membrane area required, and the like) accompanied by a careful check of the design parameters needed to see if they are known with sufficient precision to allow accurate preliminary design. For example, until quite recently it was not realized that the diffusion coefficient of urea through blood is less than one-half what it is through blood plasma, a fact that bears critically upon the design of kidneys and oxygenators.

Therefore, in the process of evaluation of the concept a number of feedback loops will be involved aimed at experimental verification or experimental determination of quantities that are thought to be critical.

STAGE 2: PILOT MODEL

After a concept has been involved and subjected to theoretical analysis and supplemented by partial experimental verification as needed, the next stage would presumably be a pilot model. It is at this point that the development may well benefit by the assistance of, or intervention of, a multitechnical organization. If on the one hand, the artificial organ is something as simple as an arterial section to be tested in an experimental animal, the group that evolves the biomaterial from which the arterial sections were made could submit it to a clinical group for evaluation. On the other hand, if one is considering a system such as an artificial kidney, with its catheters, connecting tubing, pumps, dialysis tanks, heat exchangers, and so on, a number of different engineering talents and manufacturing services are needed.

Now coming into play, to a widely varying extent, are designers, draftsmen, machine shop services, assemblers, and technicians, depending upon the complexity of the devices. It is this aspect of an artificial organ and its development that is particularly worthy of close scrutiny by this task group.

STAGE 3: REPLICATING PILOT MODELS

Even assuming the first pilot model could be or, in fact, were produced in a university laboratory, if it were successful, larger numbers of identical or nearly identical units would next be required for large-scale testing in a variety of clinical situations by medical investigators working in the same area. Thus, if the services of a multitechnical organization has not already come into play in Stage 2, they are almost forced to come into play when multiple pilot models are required, unless one takes one of the following unlikely actions. One establishes a small-scale production unit within either a university department or a hospital.

Assuming that the preceding alternatives may be dismissed, the question of the multitechnical organization arises. Various alternatives propose themselves, including:

(a) Collaboration among a university group, a hospital group, and an outside profit making or nonprofit enterprise composed of specialists or technologists appropriate to the subject matter;

(b) Broad dissemination of the idea and an invitation for wide-scale implementation, a procedure that might be accomplished, for example, by RFP issued by the sponsoring Public Health Service agency; and

(c) A new form of triangular collaboration among a university, a medical school, and an internal multitechnical organization.

Examples of the first two options are known from prior experience, and in many cases have worked very effectively, though in others rather poorly. It is to the third alternative that this draft addresses itself.

2. An Example of a Multitechnical Organization in a University-Hospital Complex.

The necessity for day-to-day direction and consultation between the initiating group, the production group, and the clinical group, suggests the desirability of a multi-technical organization near the medical and university laboratories.

Within the framework of the Massachusetts Institute of Technology and the Harvard Medical School, a close but not necessarily exact model of this institution is the Instrumentation Laboratory which, despite its nominal alliance with the Department of Aeronautics, has a staff of widely varied engineering talents and distinguished specialization in electrical engineering and a variety of distinctive or unique engineering ancillaries (for example, a precision machine shop where the machinists work in spotlessly clean surgical gowns, highly skilled draftsmen, illustrators, and so on).

It is perhaps unnecessary to point out that a facility like the Instrumentation Laboratory also has a personnel office, a purchasing department, supervisory groups, inspection rooms, warehousing facilities, and many of the other features of modern industry, including the capability to deliver "a package." Yet, this kind of laboratory, organized on neither the profit nor the conventional not-for-profit basis and drawing on the staff of the university, can function in a unique way that is probably superior to any other arrangement.

Financing of artificial organ development is now, and will probably remain, almost completely under the control, through one agency or another, of the United States Public Health Service, except in limited cases in which private enterprise can identify a sufficiently great market to make it worthwhile to risk capital and to carry development up to a significant point of progress. The history of the Dow Chemical Company hollow fiber kidney illustrates a development with industrial ramifications that make it possible to justify mounting the considerable research that Dow did in fact use in establishing its kidney program. The magnitude of the market for a specific artificial organ usually involves material production insignificant to American industry as a whole. For example, if indefinite money were available to supply an artificial kidney to every uremic patient in the United States in need of chronic dialysis, the total amount of cellophane required per year would probably be less than one day's production by the Visking Division of Union Carbide. It is, therefore, not surprising that the industrial giants of the United States are not enthusiastic about entering the field of artificial organs, except under special conditions, a pertinent one being that in undertaking this kind of work their staff may derive a considerable educational benefit and generate ideas that are applicable to nonmedical areas. It is probably the smaller and recently formed consulting or venture company that is inclined to devote a portion of its total effort to contract research on artificial organs, because the direct benefit of involvement in a growing technology will have much more effect on its staff relative to its future productivity. Indeed, it is possible to identify with the hindsight of experience various small companies that successfully specialize in certain kinds of artificial organs or ancillary equipment.

These companies, in general, are small enough so that despite the smallness of the market, the degree of specialization, and their own size make it worthwhile financially for them to operate. However, on balance, the economic aspect of artificial organ development, the probable future source of funds for development, and the order of magnitude of the effort involved focus attention on an organization *like* the Instrumentation Laboratory rather than a corporate giant in private industry.

3. Several Considerations Regarding Staffing and Operating a Development Team Consisting of University Departments, a Multitechnical Organization, and Medical School-Hospital Complex

Some interesting problems present themselves in connection with the philosophy, indeed the psychology, of an operation such as that contemplated. Two major headings are here discussed: (a) personnel, and (b) educational "pay-off."

PERSONNEL

Bluntly, there must be something in an association to attract those who become associated with it. If not high salaries, then prestige, increased reputation, the chance for promotion, the opportunity to be the first to publish or be considered a coequal in an important team, and so on.

A host of problems are raised on the subject of recompense (aside from investment opportunities, and the like). For example, the graduating chemical engineer with no industrial experience is currently (1968) being offered more than $15,000 per year, whereas the postdoctoral M.D. as a trainee may be lucky to get $7,000 under an N.I.H. Grant. It would not be wise, however, to upset straight away the financial system operative in the junior ranks of the medical profession.

To a considerable extent a university department and multitechnical group like the Instrumentation Laboratory are competing with private industry for the same intelligent, highly motivated scientists and engineers, the people with genuine creativity. Thus, the financial recompense must also compete with industry. It is not enough to argue that because the work is more interesting or important to humanity or something else that personnel entering it should be less well paid than elsewhere in our society, especially if the engineer can find the opportunity to work on interesting medical engineering problems *within* industry. It will certainly make trouble to pay different kinds of professional people (e.g., the new M.D. physician and the recent post-Ph.D. engineer) different rates, and this will be a major problem in bringing together the medical profession and the engineering profession at the junior levels in a single organization.

Again in respect to motivation, while it is desirable, and ultimately necessary, to carry out wide scale production and wide scale testing of any new artificial organ, there is a peculiar danger in rushing into widespread dissemination of a particular material or device in order to test it among widely different groups scattered around the nation. For if clinical investigators are under the impression that they are carrying out work that may be published by some other group before them —in other words, if they don't, for at least a brief period of time, have some exclusive right to investigate, they may well decline to undertake any work along these lines, instead preferring to devote their energies to problems they can evolve through their own creation and get credit for doing it. Thus, a peculiarly delicate function of triangular consortiums of the type proposed is the one that determines at what stage one releases pilot models for testing and to which clinical groups. A compelling reason for considering a triangular arrangement is that problems may be reduced to one city and two educational institutions, rather than having a large number of groups, of different calibers and widely separated from each other. Also, the top administration can quickly identify the most likely investigators in the university or the medical school-hospital complex to assist in development or evaluation.

EDUCATIONAL "PAY-OFF":

If the kind of operation sketched above is to have real meaning either for the medical school-hospital complex or for the university, it must, to a significant degree, accomplish the following:

(1) Feedback into the educational process, directly involving the students at both the graduate and undergraduate levels in the university, the academic staff and other professional personnel, and the various ranks of medicine from the chief of service through the interns to the third and fourth year medical school students.

(2) This implies not only education but money may be fed back into the university and into the hospital for ancillary and new basic research. The cost of this should be taken as overhead to the total cost of the operation

and should be computed as such. For example, twenty percent of the direct cost of a development would be alloted for education and basic research in universities and hospitals outside the multitechnical organization. (The figure of twenty percent could vary in either direction, of course.) It seems self-evident that if the multitechnical organization is so far removed from the university or from the hospital complex that interchange of people and ideas is made difficult, then the proposal would be reduced to considering the placing of a development task in the hands of any kind of qualified group organized either on a profit or nonprofit basis.

Letter of July 29, 1968 from Edwin W. Salzman, M.D., Associate Director of Surgery, Beth Israel Hospital, to Professor Edward W. Merrill.

I have reviewed with some care your document on a Task Force Committee on Artificial Organs. It strikes me as being a well-balanced piece of work. There are several points that deserve emphasis and that seem particularly worthy of detail.

The advantage of a joint effort as opposed to a unilateral effort seems to be to allow one to capitalize on the rather disparate strengths of separate disciplines for a common purpose. It seems an efficient way for product development although not necessarily for the advancement of knowledge. Cross-fertilization and fresh insights are obvious benefits. In addition, the prospect of breeding a new variety of individual with a foot in each camp seems desirable, and I should think that a joint effort would be educational for engineering students as well as for fledgling biologists. A point which is seldom appreciated is the way in which such a joint effort upgrades biological sciences by forcing upon them physical and mathematical techniques that otherwise are too little used. By requiring the biologist to think in quantitative terms such a situation uncovers voids in his knowledge and exposes areas of ignorance that might otherwise be allowed to lie dormant.

I'm not sure that such a joint effort lends itself to basic "conceptual" nonapplied research. Administrative problems may make such an arrangement unwieldy and there is, of course, the awkward salary structure that you mention. Frequent and detailed reviews of the performance of each side by the other strike me as being vital for the success of such an arrangement. The alternative is a series of costly and inefficient misconceptions. One must also guard against a threat to established collaborations at the individual level, such as the one that we have enjoyed so much ourselves. It would be important not to divert funds or facilities from such personal relationships which are likely to remain fruitful, particularly in investigation that is not clearly product-directed.

Thank you for the opportunity to review this paper.

Task Group Report on Bioengineering Curricula

Murray Eden
PROFESSOR OF ELECTRICAL ENGINEERING
MASSACHUSETTS INSTITUTE OF TECHNOLOGY, CHAIRMAN

Frederick Abernathy
ASSOCIATE DEAN OF THE DIVISION OF ENGINEERING AND APPLIED PHYSICS
HARVARD UNIVERSITY

W. Gerald Austen
PROFESSOR OF SURGERY
HARVARD MEDICAL SCHOOL

Raymond F. Baddour
PROFESSOR OF CHEMICAL ENGINEERING
MASSACHUSETTS INSTITUTE OF TECHNOLOGY

Gordon S. Brown
DEAN OF THE SCHOOL OF ENGINEERING
MASSACHUSETTS INSTITUTE OF TECHNOLOGY

Paul E. Brown
EXECUTIVE OFFICER OF THE CENTER FOR
ADVANCED ENGINEERING STUDY
MASSACHUSETTS INSTITUTE OF TECHNOLOGY

Gordon L. Brownell
APPLIED PHYSICIST, MEDICINE
MASSACHUSETTS GENERAL HOSPITAL

Edward J. Burger
DEPARTMENT OF PHYSIOLOGY
HARVARD SCHOOL OF PUBLIC HEALTH

Philip A. Drinker
LECTURER IN MECHANICAL ENGINEERING
MASSACHUSETTS INSTITUTE OF TECHNOLOGY

Melvin J. Glimcher
Judith M. Ashley
PROFESSOR OF ORTHOPEDIC SURGERY
MASSACHUSETTS GENERAL HOSPITAL

Peter Katona
ASSISTANT PROFESSOR OF ELECTRICAL ENGINEERING
MASSACHUSETTS INSTITUTE OF TECHNOLOGY

Robert W. Mann
PROFESSOR OF MECHANICAL ENGINEERING
MASSACHUSETTS INSTITUTE OF TECHNOLOGY

Sanford A. Miller
ASSOCIATE PROFESSOR OF NUTRITION
MASSACHUSETTS INSTITUTE OF TECHNOLOGY

William T. Peake
ASSOCIATE PROFESSOR OF ELECTRICAL ENGINEERING
MASSACHUSETTS INSTITUTE OF TECHNOLOGY

Walter A. Rosenblith
PROFESSOR OF ELECTRICAL ENGINEERING, CHAIRMAN OF THE FACULTY
MASSACHUSETTS INSTITUTE OF TECHNOLOGY

David D. Rutstein
RIDLEY WATTS PROFESSOR OF PREVENTIVE MEDICINE
HARVARD MEDICAL SCHOOL

Albert O. Seeler
HEAD OF THE MEDICAL DEPARTMENT
MASSACHUSETTS INSTITUTE OF TECHNOLOGY

William M. Siebert
PROFESSOR OF ELECTRICAL ENGINEERING
MASSACHUSETTS INSTITUTE OF TECHNOLOGY

Ascher H. Shapiro
CHAIRMAN OF THE DEPARTMENT OF MECHANICAL ENGINEERING
MASSACHUSETTS INSTITUTE OF TECHNOLOGY

Irwin W. Sizer
DEAN OF THE GRADUATE SCHOOL
MASSACHUSETTS INSTITUTE OF TECHNOLOGY

Benson R. Snyder
PSYCHIATRIST IN CHIEF
MEDICAL DEPARTMENT
MASSACHUSETTS INSTITUTE OF TECHNOLOGY

Louis D. Smullin
CHAIRMAN OF THE DEPARTMENT OF ELECTRICAL ENGINEERING
MASSACHUSETTS INSTITUTE OF TECHNOLOGY

Richard J. Wurtman
ASSOCIATE PROFESSOR OF NUTRITION
MASSACHUSETTS INSTITUTE OF TECHNOLOGY

Laurence R. Young
ASSOCIATE PROFESSOR OF AERONAUTICS
MASSACHUSETTS INSTITUTE OF TECHNOLOGY

Jerrold R. Zacharias
INSTITUTE PROFESSOR, PHYSICS
MASSACHUSETTS INSTITUTE OF TECHNOLOGY

The task of this committee is to consider ways to improve the education of students who intend to pursue careers in which the physical sciences, engineering, and mathematics will serve as substantial parts of their intellectual foundation, but who will apply their skills in the development of biological knowledge, the practice of medicine, and in the service of better medical and health care.

So broad a charge covers a variety of different careers. We have partitioned this set into six different categories.

1. Graduate students who intend to prepare themselves for careers as engineers or applied physical scientists and who will also work in areas of biology and medicine.

2. Graduate engineers in engineering, physics, mathematics, industrial management, and so on, whose research interests have turned to specific areas of biology and medicine.

3. Undergraduates who intend to go on to medical school.

4. Medical school students who wish to enhance their backgrounds in the physical sciences and technology and who wish to spend their elective time in medical specialties for which such educational backgrounds will be valuable adjuncts to classical medical education.

5. Post-M.D. students who intend to pursue research careers.

6. Physicians in practice who wish to learn enough about new technological and analytic tools to improve and sharpen their skills in medical practice.

Clearly, because these groups have widely different motivations, they must be considered separately. Perhaps our competences and backgrounds are not adequate for providing thoughtful and informed answers at this time. However, some suggestions for the training of the latter three categories have been considered by the task group on continuing education. Therefore, we would like to comment primarily on educational questions relative to the first three categories.

First, with respect to undergraduates who seek to go on to medical school, the ad hoc education subcommittee of the Harvard-M.I.T. Joint Committee on Engineering and Living Systems has recommended an experimental program that would involve interdigitation of the academic work in the undergraduate school and the Harvard Medical School. Informal discussions concerning questions of curriculum have been held with five academic departments at M.I.T.: biology, electrical engineering, mechanical engineering, chemical engineering, and aeronautics and astronautics.

It appears that in each of these cases a student would find it possible both to acquire the fundamentals of the relevant discipline and to satisfy the formal requirements for admission to medical school without subjecting himself to an unduly heavy course load. But perhaps more important than the matter of the formal course work, each student would be under the guidance of a tutorial committee drawn from both schools. In this way, the student's academic career could be modified to accord with his unique needs and interests. This experimental program, while still a significant first step, cannot be regarded as more than transitional. With the possible exception of certain special seminars, the formal curriculum will be made up of existing subjects. Indeed, any undergraduate could now follow such a curriculum under existing departmental practices. Eventually an interdigitated B.S.-M.D. program could be established under which M.I.T. and Harvard Medical School would grant credit for appropriate work done at each institution.

Concerning the education of graduate students who come to this area with a foundation in engineering, applied mathematics, or management, we would merely observe that there are already a substantial number of graduate students doing thesis research in medical or health related areas who have not encountered serious administrative obstacles in their paths. This is not to say that there is no room for improvement in the mechanism for handling such students or that there is no need for interdepartmental committees to modify existing procedures or requirements that deal with qualifying examinations, formal curricula, or even admissions. Nevertheless, it appears that there are very few, if any, faculty who feel that this aspect of the educational process deserves much of our attention at this point.

Finally, on every occasion in the last five years when

the question of biomedical engineering education has been raised at M.I.T., there has been almost unanimous agreement that we regard it as essential that the student be educated to competence and mastery in one of the existing engineering or scientific fields. Thus, every graduate receiving an Sc.D., for example, in chemical engineering, must be a well trained chemical engineer even though his research may have dealt with the solution of a problem deriving its interest from the peculiar requirements of biological application. There is, in other words, no such thing as a biomedical engineer. There is probably not even such a thing as a biomedical chemical engineer or biomedical mechanical engineer. To consider an example, a student prepared and interested in problems of the flow of biological fluids will be prepared differently—from the point of view of both mechanical engineering and biology—from a student who concerned with nervous control of a mechanical substitute of a particular muscle. If one accepts this view, it is clearly inappropriate to suggest a special curriculum in biomedical engineering.

As a matter of fact, so far as graduate students are concerned, one can hardly talk of a single curriculum in say, electrical engineering; each student's formal course work, and indeed the other aspects of his academic career, are in large measure unique to him. So far as biological and medical course work is concerned, it is already possible for any student to cross register between the two academic institutions cooperating in this program. Where then are the problems?

The fundamental problem is the lack of courses in biology and the health sciences that are taught in a way appropriate to the style and philosophy of the quantitative sciences. It has become increasingly clear that despite the felt need for engineering methodologies and concepts on the part of many interested and creative people in the life sciences, and despite the desire for collaborative efforts with the physical sciences to enrich the productivity and the depth of such biological sciences, very little in the way of specific and substantive suggestions for future work has emerged from discussions on the subject. The reason for this seems to be uncertainty and unfamiliarity with what the engineering disciplines have to offer the life sciences (above and beyond the intuitive understanding that such offerings are bound to be valuable).

In keeping with this concept, let us express the opinion that it is now appropriate to try to develop an attitude toward biology and medicine in which mathematics, physics, and engineering methodologies are as much significant foundational elements as anatomy, biochemistry and physiology. It has been suggested in the past that such treatment of physics and mathematics should be of a fundamentally different nature if the goal is to develop them as the background for the life sciences. This is a more radical suggestion, perhaps, than would be acceptable to most members of the faculty, but the treatment of the life sciences needs substantial redefinition if both M.I.T. and Harvard are to move in the direction of the goal set forth. However, the principal educational interests of the life sciences and health related departments at both schools is clearly different, and it would be unrealistic to expect them to develop subject matter for a series of academic offerings in a way that would be, from their point of view, much in the nature of service courses.

But it is clear that to prepare students for work involving a close mesh between the physical sciences and biology, a change in the traditional modes of presentation in teaching the life sciences is needed. One approach that might be fruitful would involve a shift toward the use of engineering concepts for the basic approach and orientation for special courses in anatomy, physiology, and so on. To take some examples, one might study many aspects of functional anatomy from the standpoint of the mechanics of statics, carefully noting the mechanical significance of structural arrangements in the skeletal and locomotor system. Perhaps the study of control systems could form the unitary concept for a new approach to the teaching of physiology. Each functional unit in the living system could be looked at as a regulatory mechanism, and the abstract study of automatic regulation and its attendant engineering techniques could be the basis for such a program.

Alternatively, certain disciplines could be presented from several different points of view. For example, neurophysiology could be given first by an electrical engineer active in this area, then by a molecular biologist, and perhaps again by a communications scientist. Each unit would be a consistent and penetrating presentation of the important techniques and results. In this way, it is hoped that the student would not only benefit from the variety of viewpoints but learn important, generally applicable analytic techniques at the same time.

Equally necessary is a biological complement to the engineering curriculum. Just as the biologist should become schooled in quantitative modes of reasoning, so must the engineer and physical scientist be introduced to those peculiar features of the biologist's thinking that are necessary for meaningful collaboration. Such a commonplace biological concept as the hierarchy of structure in anatomy (subcellular, cellular, tissue, organ, organism) cannot be truly said to be part of a physical scientist's background. These scientists must also become accustomed to the problems of biologic variation in their subjects, learn to recognize priorities for the organism in a complex of structures and functions, and recognize the immense potential for change and adaptation under a wide variety of conditions. In addition to this, a series of seminars or courses designed to orient nonphysicians to the clinical aspects of the life sciences could be especially fruitful in educating engineers in the biomedical area and interesting them in new research.

At this point, however, it is clear that there are a number of major unsolved problems. Some kind of reorganization in training is probably necessary if concepts and methodologies from mathematics and the physical sciences are to be successfully applied in the areas of biology and health care, and vice versa. Although there are already established routines and working relations, the desired results can only be obtained through experimentation. Some significant and innovative steps, short of a disruptive crash program, can be taken now to begin the evolution of a satisfactory educational structure.

Therefore, we would like to offer for your consideration and criticism a set of three parallel initiatives. First, that a faculty group be constituted to produce concrete proposals, using the following method of attack. Several specific research goals compatible with the interests of the group would be examined in detail, with a view to detailing the basic disciplines considered fundamental to a worker wishing to involve himself in this area. By way of illustration, such a group might take the problem of pattern recognition in blood smears. Besides his skills in electrical engineering and computer science, a student wishing to enter this research area would need to have some knowledge of the physical and organic chemistry of staining reactions, a good foundation in cellular physiology and pathology, and perhaps some background in clinical hematology. Or again, the study of control in biochemical processes on the cellular level could be examined. Besides the engineering skills necessary for control systems theory, cellular physiology, enzyme kinetics, and physical and organic chemistry are some obvious prerequisites. When a number of such preliminary patterns have been worked out, there is bound to result at least, a better "feel" for the problem and its implications; and at the very best, we may even be able to advance some substantive proposals that are both innovative and practical.

Second, we would recommend that a group of students soon begin work with a tutorial committee who will guide them in choosing subjects appropriate to their interests. In this way, we shall be better able to study the processes involved in training individuals interested in biomedical engineering problems and thereby be better equipped to deal with an area in which so many of the problems are as yet unforeseen.

Finally, it would be desirable to have several of the life scientists engaged in these projects (e.g., an anatomist, a biochemist, a pharmacologist and a physiologist) devote a substantial portion of their time (a semester or more) to the problem of adapting the training of their disciplines to the needs of the special kinds of students about whom we have been talking. The recommendation is, therefore, that a body be established, and appropriately funded, to take on the responsibility of carrying out these tasks.

Task Group Report on Biological Control Systems

Richard J. Wurtman
ASSOCIATE PROFESSOR OF NUTRITION
MASSACHUSETTS INSTITUTE OF TECHNOLOGY, CHAIRMAN

Donald Gann
CASE-WESTERN RESERVE

Dr. Sidney Lees
CHAIRMAN, BIOENGINEERING DEPARTMENT
FORSYTHE DENTAL CENTER

Dr. Gardner Quarton
NEUROSCIENCES RESEARCH PROGRAM

Biological regulatory mechanisms operate on at least two levels of organization in mammals; the controlled function may be the concentration of a compound (or the rate at which it changes) within a cell or it may be a characteristic of the extracellular fluid (e.g., temperature, osmolality, pH, cortisol concentration). Many of the exciting and important advances in biomedical sciences made during the past few decades have concerned the former; i.e., intracellular type of regulation; such concepts as enzyme induction and activation, end-product inhibition, and metabolic compartments have enriched the whole of theoretical biology and provided much of the intellectual underpinning for current biological research. Unfortunately, intracellular regulatory mechanisms in intact mammals are usually difficult to monitor and tend to be even more difficult to manipulate. Changes in the levels of key substances are considerably easier to follow in mammalian extracellular fluid, and the levels can usually be manipulated at will. One has only to contrast the relative ease of measuring the calcium concentration or temperature of the blood to measuring the calcium or temperature within cells in order to come to this conclusion. The components of the systems that control parameters in the extracellular fluid are relatively easy to isolate, and the systems themselves often show important structural similarities. For example, the regulatory loops controlling the concentrations of glucose, water, and cortisol in extracellular fluid all utilize cerebral sensors, neuroendocrine transducers, and distant effector organs. For these reasons, it is suggested that the regulation of the extracellular fluid in humans and other mammals constitutes a promising area for collaborative study by engineers and biologists.

The following report describes several projects in which engineering knowledge could be profitably utilized to approach the regulation of the extracellular fluid. We are interested in working on these projects and are currently involved with some of them. In preparing this report, we have been aided by half a dozen members of the M.I.T. staff and the Boston medical community, who graciously provided criticism and a sounding-board. We were unable to obtain specific suggestions as to additional projects from most of the people we contacted; all believed that engineering concepts and techniques had enormous contributions to make to the study of biological regulatory systems, but none could identify specific problems not already under investigation that might utilize this approach.

This absence of ideas among creative and interested people leads us to suspect that (a) most biologists— even at M.I.T.—have only a remote knowledge of engineering concepts and techniques and do not know how to use what is available to them; and (b) very few biologists think of regulation in the body in other than the most simple terms. If all extracellular regulatory mechanisms utilized only simple closed feedback loops and maintained constant levels which are independent of time, there would be little need for the engineer in theoretical biology. A lot has happened since Claude Bernard.

We would first propose that the National Academy of Engineering organize a program specifically designed to foster the growth of the study of mammalian regulatory biology and to encourage engineers to contribute to this growth. Engineers and regulatory biologists should be brought together to educate each other about their respective fields. The engineers could explain what they mean by "control systems" and "regulation," describe the common structural components of such systems, tell how they go about studying their dynamic properties, explain how they model control systems, and so forth. The biologists could tell what is known about the regulation of each of the thirty or forty controlled parameters in the extracellular fluid. The engineers could encourage the biologists to abstract, to simplify, and to isolate the components of their systems; the biologists could force the engineers to stay close to the natures of the matters in question. Out of such meetings might come, perhaps, innovative courses at several levels (i.e., for teachers and for students), and possibly even the basis of undergraduate or graduate bioengineering curricula at M.I.T. Clearly, such meetings—and only such meetings—will spawn reasonable research projects. They could take place on a continuing basis at an appropriate center on the M.I.T. campus.

It is general practice in mammalian physiology (and even in clinical medicine) for the investigator to assume that regulated functions in the extracellular fluid do not change with time; hence it is permissable to sample a function under study only once each day and at any time that happens to be convenient. This assumption is born of necessity, as it is usually not possible to do otherwise except at the price of multiple venepunctures and great inconvenience to investigator and investigated. Where it has been possible to obtain multiple measurements of regulated functions at different times of day (as, for example, of body temperature) it has been well documented that this assumption of constancy is not supported by the data: "Normal" body temperature may be 97.6°F at 7:00 A.M. and 99.2°F at 5:00 P.M.; and early in the morning 98.6°F may be evidence of a fever. Telemetric devices are now available which allow body temperature to be measured repeatedly in the undisturbed animal or human.

Similar devices should be developed, if possible, to transmit information about regulated chemical functions, including pH, osmolality, ion concentrations, and the like. Such information could add a new dimension —that of time—to our understanding of bodily physiology. It may also provide insights into pathophysiology and aids to diagnosis. Ultimately, such devices could be coupled with artificial effectors like the cardiac pacemaker.

Pharmacologists and organic chemists now synthesize large numbers of new compounds, many of which have never before existed. It becomes increasingly important that large-scale methods be developed for screening these compounds for toxic as well as therapeutic effects. Current screening methods, which use small groups of laboratory animals, are inadequate for this purpose. It would be of great use if lines of human cells could be grown in tissue culture whose responses to added chemicals would be genuinely predictive of the *in vivo* responses of their organs of origin. To date, it has not been possible to develop such cell lines. Tissue culture cells are adequate for certain virologic and biochemical problems, but they have contributed little to pharmacology or toxicology.

One reason for this inadequacy may relate to the fact that our knowledge of the chemical milieu in which these cells exist *in vivo* (i.e., surrounded by extracellular fluid) has not been used to full advantage in designing

96

their *in vitro* media. Scientists who grow cells in tissue culture take pains to control the concentrations of water, sodium, glucose, and perhaps twenty-odd other chemicals (most recently, oxygen) in their media. However, they fail to worry about an equivalent number of other compounds that are always present in extracellular fluid and whose concentrations are normally regulated and kept within a narrow range. A large-scale project should be undertaken to develop the desired cell lines, with the following phases:

1. Let regulatory biologists consider all the chemicals that are always available to cells *in vivo* in regulated concentrations. Together with engineers, they should devise means of controlling these compounds in tissue culture media, determining which are really necessary to maintain the biochemical integrity of the cells, in what concentrations, and so forth.

2. Pharmacologists and cell biologists should jointly characterize enzyme systems that might be used to predict the responses of these cells (and their organs of origin) to various chemical agents.

We hope to initiate pilot studies toward these goals when time and funds become available.

Appendix 1

After this report was written, I had an opportunity to speak with Professor Donald Gann, Director of the Biomedical Engineering Center at the Case-Western Reserve School of Medicine, about his group's plans for work in biological regulatory mechanisms. He stated that several months ago they had set up a task force to make recommendations for specific research projects in this area. The task force proved unsuccessful and was disbanded after a month or two. He attributes its lack of success to his difficulty in finding biologists with an understanding of the philosophy of engineering to appoint to it. Task forces set up to plan development-type projects (e.g., telemetry, artificial hearts) had a clearer mandate and were, on the whole, more successful. Ultimately, Dr. Gann set up a research program on biological regulatory mechanisms that was concerned with his own ideas and research interests. They are described below. Dr. Gann thinks that there are perhaps a half a dozen biologists in the country with the training and ability to make important contributions to this area; he hopes to bring them all to Case-Western Reserve. His program consists of three projects:

1. A study on neural and endocrine factors that regulate the cardiovascular apparatus: he hopes to model the circulatory system.

2. A study of the interactions between adjacent neurons grown in tissue culture: he hopes these interactions can simulate transfer in the body.

3. An application of membrane biophysics to the study of transport physiology.

These programs are just now being initiated. Their fates may provide useful data to the M.I.T.-Harvard project and may aid in the selection of local goals.

Appendix 2

Dr. John B. Stanbury, of the M.I.T. Department of Nutrition and Food Science, contributed the following list of specific projects that might utilize engineering approaches in studying biological regulatory mechanisms.

1. Engineering of tissue culture techniques for production of peptide and other hormones, especially GH, ACTH, TSH, and releasing factors. These might be used for therapeutic purposes, diagnostic tests, and specific labeling for physiological studies.

2. Development of laser beam scanners for scanning poly-acrylamide gells at 260, 280, and 620μ

3. Automation of radioimmunoassay, resin displacement, and photofluorometry steroid techniques.

4. Application of engineering procedures for automating specimen preparation for electron microscopy.

5. Biological control systems modeling and analysis by computer, such as thyroid and adrenal systems.

6. Monitoring of blood pressure by ultrasound.

7. Microengineering of enzyme systems for implantation in the body behind semipermeable walls, e.g., urea cycle enzymes, aspartase, and phenylalanine hydroxylase.

8. Model control systems in tissue culture: pituitary-thyroid, pituitary-adrenal, hypothalamus-pituitary-thyroid (tissue separation by millipore barriers).

9. General study of the pulsatile systems of the body: cardiac rhythmicity, brain rhythmicity, drug effects on mechanism of pulsing chemical systems, pulsing membrane charges.

10. Scanning techniques:
Regional flow in the brain, liver, and thyroid, using short-lived isotopes and lag-time camera scanning.[123]

Appendix 3:
THE STUDY OF MAMMALIAN PHYSIOLOGY USING BIOTELEMETRY TECH-NOLOGY. EXCERPTS FROM A COLLABORATIVE PROPOSAL OF THE DRAPER LABORATORY AND THE DEPARTMENTS OF FOOD AND NUTRITION AND CHEMICAL ENGINEERING

INTRODUCTION

The study of mammalian physiology is markedly restricted by the near impossibility of making continuous measurements of most bodily functions in human beings and experimental animals. Almost all the information currently available about "normal levels" of compounds in blood or tissues or "normal rates" at which processes occur derives from experiments in which a given subject or animal was sampled only once, or at most four or five times, in a twenty-four-hour period. So it is not surprising that homeostasis remains the dominant general theory of how the body works. When physiologists begin to study the regulation of a particular rate or level, they commonly assume that the function being examined normally shows only minor variations from its set point. Since "normal levels" exist are independent of time, the physiologist believes it permissible to measure blood calcium in humans or tissue enzyme activities at any moment convenient to him, because he assumes that whenever these functions are sampled, the same values will obtain. The persistence of this view of physiology is understandable inasmuch as the physiologist or clinician most commonly has no choice but to sample once and pray for constancy. However, it becomes less and less supportable as evidence accumulates that most functions in the body are, in fact, quite different depending on the time of day they are measured. At all three levels of physiologic regulation (intracellular, extracellular, behavioral) bodily functions have been identified that vary markedly with the time of day. It has become abundantly clear that functions not dependent on the time of day constitute the exceptions in bodily physiology.

Hence, it is essential that techniques be devised that allow physiologic functions to be monitored continually. Ideally, these techniques should leave the subject or animal undisturbed; nor should they restrict his activity or otherwise modify his behavior. To achieve these goals, several laboratories have, during the past few decades, attempted to construct telemetric devices. These devices contain a sensor, which converts a measurement of the function under study to an electrical signal, and a radio transmitter. A radio receiver is kept at a distance from the subject or experimental animal; this converts the signal from the telemeter into data that can be recorded and analyzed.

Both the sensors and the radio transmitters now in use have drawbacks: to date, it has been possible to construct usable sensors only for physical functions (e.g., temperature, pressure, waveforms); telemeters have not been developed that can obtain continuous measurements of, for example, blood sodium or calcium concentrations. Moreover, the transmitters generally use batteries; this adds to their bulk and often precludes implantation within body spaces that should be studied (e.g., within the cranial cavity); and it necessitates frequent recalibrations inasmuch as the batteries tend to run down.

We have initiated a project whose long-term goal is the development of telemetric devices which can obtain continuous measurements on a wide variety of bodily functions. As such devices become available, we hope to obtain fundamental information about the ways that biochemical and physical phenomena in the body vary during the course of a day. These data can be useful in obtaining a more accurate understanding of normal bodily physiology, enhancing our ability to recognize abnormal levels and rates and thus to diagnose disease states, and increasing the effectiveness of treatment regimens. For example, it is widely held but poorly documented that patients suffering from severe cardiovascular disease show a greater tendency to die at night than would be expected on the basis of chance alone. This tendency may be related to another poorly defined phenomenon, the tendency of blood pressure and sympathetic nervous tone to decrease at night. It seems likely, though it is as yet unproved, that certain drugs given to critically ill patients to maintain blood pressure are less effective at night than during daylight hours. (This seems especially likely in the case of agents like metaraminol, which act by liberating bound norepinephrine from sympathetic nerve endings.) To define the time-dependence of blood pressure regulation would be most useful in monitoring blood pressure continuously in normal subjects and patients. Measurements could be obtained first in the untreated person and again following the administration of agents to raise blood pressure. A demonstration that the response of blood pressure to a given dose of a drug differed at 4:00 A.M. from that seen at 4:00 P.M. could have important implications for medical practice. Many additional examples could be cited from physiology and clinical medicine to justify the potential importance of continuous physiological monitoring with telemeters. We propose to expand our pilot project as follows:

1. We wish to construct an apparatus for receiving telemetric signals and for recording and analyzing their content of information. This apparatus will at first be used in association with temperature-sensitive telemeters that are already in operation; it will be designed to record signals from telemeters sensitive to several different physiological functions (e.g., temperature, pressure, plasma calcium, electroencephalographic waves, etc.) in the same animal.

2. We hope to obtain fundamental information about the control of the daily rhythm in bodily temperature. Using the system described above, we will ask such questions as the following: Is the signal responsible for the temperature rhythm generated exogenously (i.e., outside the animal, as by the daily light cycle) or endogenously? If endogenously, can it be localized to a particular brain area or network by lesions or by pharmacologic manipulations? Does the expression of this rhythm require the activity of various endocrine organs? Is it dependent upon the ingestion of protein? Do antipyretic agents (e.g., aspirin) lower body temperature in normal afebrile subjects at the time of the daily temperature peak? If not, how is a temperature of 99.0°F in a normal person (i.e., at 4:00 P.M.) differentiated from the same temperature in a patient with fever (i.e., at 7:00 A.M.)?

3. In collaboration with other departments of M.I.T. we hope to develop sensors that respond to biochemical functions (e.g., blood pH, calcium concentration, glucose level) and that can be coupled with telemetric transmitters.

PRESENT STATUS OF BIOTELEMETRY AT M.I.T.

A number of implantable, temperature-sensing telemeters of the thermistor-blocking-oscillator type have been constructed for the study of circadian temperature rhythms in laboratory rats. A variety of receiving antennas for use with these telemeters were built and tested, and a modest system for recording telemetric data from up to ten cages was installed. Considerable output, in the form of printed paper tape, has been obtained to date.

Experience has also been gained with a commercially available system using FM termperature telemeters. These systems have emphasized the need and direction of future development in the biomedical-telemetry area.

Experience with commercially available units have shown that their performance, reliability, and size are incompatible with the objectives of a research effort directed at physiological monitoring using implantable telemeters. Much work can and should be done to improve the stability, reliability, and output characteristics and also reduce the size and energy drain associated with existing telemeters.

Even the simple system utilized to date proves the need for an adequate, reliable data-handling system. The simple ten-cage system produced more than 1,400 distinct pieces of raw data per day, making hand data reduction a sizable task.

ESTIMATED COST

The estimated cost of this program is $468,400. Of this, $204,800 would be used the first year and $131,800 for each of the next two years.

Task Group Report on Continuing Education

Paul E. Brown
EXECUTIVE OFFICER, CENTER FOR ADVANCED ENGINEERING STUDY
MASSACHUSETTS INSTITUTE OF TECHNOLOGY, CO-CHAIRMAN

Daniel D. Federman
ASSISTANT DEAN FOR CONTINUING EDUCATION
HARVARD MEDICAL SCHOOL AND
ASSOCIATE PHYSICIAN AND CHIEF OF THE UNIT ON EDUCATION
MASSACHUSETTS GENERAL HOSPITAL, CO-CHAIRMAN

Medical science is changing at a very rapid rate. Physicians, medical scientists and biomedical engineers, because of their educational backgrounds and the nature of their work, are oriented toward keeping abreast of new developments. However, it is often not possible with present methods for practicing physicians to learn all they should about the latest methods of preventing, detecting, and treating disease, or for medical researchers to learn as much as they should about disciplines that are outside but relevant to their own. More effective ways must be found to make knowledge concerning new developments available to those who need it. This may vary from state-of-the-art information in an individual's own field to more basic concepts in another field that can provide insights that lead to problem solutions.

The groups to be considered include: practicing physicians; a special group best represented by the term "Directors of Medical Education" (DME); medical school and engineering faculty members; and young research workers in either field. These people are so diverse in their needs and preparation that they will be considered separately.

Practicing Physicians

From the viewpoint of the American public, the continuing education of physicians is perhaps the most important single topic. Physicians are in short supply now, a condition that will worsen in the coming years. This means, among other things, that physicians can keep busy (and therefore well paid) without having to be good at their work or to keep well informed by modern standards. Although recent judicial precedents and legislation are beginning to change this tradition, the entrepreneurial independence of the physicians has not yet been overcome. Thus, educational programs aimed at him must be economical in their use of his time and imaginative in taking advantage of his motivation.

A practical plan for continuing education for the practicing physician might consist of several parts. A minimum basic program would consist of ward rounds with his peers and available house staff and weekly formal sessions, such as grand rounds, clinicopathological conferences, occasional didactic lectures, journal reviews, etc. The Department of Continuing Education at Harvard Medical School is now beginning an active collaboration with community hospitals to introdue and foster such programs. In addition to such *in situ* activities, however, the practicing physician should have intermittent "refresher" programs. These are currently arranged by medical societies, specialty groups, or academic institutions, and although such programs are not optimally planned, there are many of them available.

The M.I.T.-Harvard Medical School collaboration is necessary for planning significant advances in these programs. First, there should be a study of the motivation of practicing physicians for undertaking continuing education programs. This investigation should not only examine current problems but should also use emerging communications technology, both for acquiring its data and as a subject of study. That is, the study should outline specific ways in which the new instrumentation and communications methods could change the requirements of the physician for a program of self-education and improve its appeal to him.

Second, there should be a feasibility study. Much has been made of the role of television and two-way radio links in doctor education. These have generally started well but have not endured. A major criticism has been that the doctor-student's role is too passive and that much of the material is not relevant to his needs. The new technology would seem to have promise on two scores. Programmed learning techniques, including simulation and pattern recognition, might serve to make the student more active. M.I.T.-Harvard cooperation could be enlisted in preparing teaching materials for home or hospital-based study. The study could focus on new cues for delimiting the doctor's effective knowledge (i.e., intellectual boundary setting) and new methods of getting him in contact with the current needed information. The latter might include computer-assisted analysis of the data in a difficult case; symptom-cued retrieval from a bank of information pertinent to the clinical problems; or symptom-cued simulation of the clinical problem with prompt generation of a problem set, within which the physician could solve for either a diagnosis or an approach applicable to his patient. The hardware and software needed for such systems will almost certainly be too expensive for community hospitals, but a feasibility study would disclose what kind of terminals or other access to the system would be useful in hospitals and communities of varying size.

The M.I.T. Center for Advanced Engineering Study is actively involved in exploring ways of making the material offered in its special subjects available for individual self-study. The self-study format includes specially written texts and notes supplemented by films, video tapes and/or audio tapes. The center has installed a television facility fully capable of producing broadcast quality programs. The center is developing graduate level self-study subjects for engineers in industry. Special texts being written are based on the experience gained in offering the subjects in the Practicing Engineer Advanced Study Program, an on-campus academic year program for experienced engineers and scientists. Lectures, keyed to the texts, are videotaped: and videotape copies are made from the original recordings for use in industry.

Studies are also needed to determine how the material can best be made available to the physician and how the physician can be motivated to make use of the material. The hospital in which the physician treats his patients might have an information center staffed and equipped to keep him informed in areas of interest to him, to provide answers to his questions (either with the help of a knowledgeable librarian or by a remote console linked to other sources of information), and to provide links between remote terminals and sophisticated diagnostic and analytic facilities. Such a center would be the place for a videotape machine or other audiovisual aids that the physician could use to view or listen to recordings, alone or with colleagues whenever convenient and useful to him. In addition to review material and subject material based on full-time study programs for physicians, scientists, and engineers, and material that evolved from offerings for medical students (below), the information center would be the repository for accurate evaluations of the very latest medical equipment and drugs.

Having such a center in every hospital is, of course, not feasible because of costs and space requirements.

Regional information centers may be a reasonable and workable compromise. Even in the vicinity of teaching hospitals there may be a need for regional information centers to match the needs of the practicing physician.

The cost of making videotape recordings will vary from one to two thousand dollars per hour (for straightforward material that can be recorded without special preparation, rehearsing, or rerecording) to ten thousand dollars per hour or more (for expertly produced recordings of laboratory procedures and programs requiring considerable preparation or development). The cost of the copies of the original tape can be estimated at about one hundred dollars per one-hour copy.

Directors of Medical Education (DME)

The DMEs can be looked on as connecting the practicing physician with the advances in medical information generated in the urban teaching centers. In the past, the DME has functioned to supervise the house staff and to plan teaching activities for the professional staff. The DME is less hindered by the limitations of time that make it impractical for the ordinary practicing physician to come for extended periods of training. We conceive of a new role for him; he would come to the university complex for intensive educational exposure aimed both at improving his fund of knowledge *and* at preparing him specifically for his role in educating his own hospital's staff. This would take several forms. We propose that the DME return for periodic educational exercises prepared for him to transmit to his hospital's staff. Objective content could be given to the process by preparing teaching materials that would be evaluated, then used at the hospitals from which the DME had come. Such materials might include videotapes, computer programs, audiotapes, short motion picture films, etc. The development of this material might be planned in a special department created by M.I.T.-Harvard Medical School. Circulation among the hospitals would lessen the need for duplication.

Close liaison between Harvard Medical School and M.I.T. would be needed for success in a program of this type. It is hoped that the DME can serve to articulate the maturing engineering and communications techniques to the point where they are ready for application in the community hospitals. But these men are not well trained in mathematics and the other requisite sciences and will need special programs designed at the university. These will in no way be comparable to those currently offered for undergraduates or returning engineering graduate students. In order to present this material properly without either absurdly diluting it or making it too abstruse, a sensitive and subtle collaboration between the faculties will be required. Neither faculty by itself will be able to provide this service.

Medical School and Engineering School Faculty Members

It is clearly impossible and impractical for large numbers of practicing physicians and medical researchers to leave their work for four to twelve months of full-time study. However, full-time study programs would influence the larger numbers in several ways. The teachers who attend would influence many students; the engineers and physicians, because of the unique interdisciplinary knowledge they would gain from the program, would be able to bridge the gap between medicine and engineering or science and become able to direct, guide, or influence the activities of their colleagues.

The M.I.T. Center for Advanced Engineering Study has pioneered in developing intensive, full-time, nondegree programs for experienced professionals from industry, government and other academic institutions. The programs of the center prepare men for future roles in: a) technical management, b) creative leadership in an area that requires the application of knowledge from several disciplines, and c) in-depth accomplishment in one discipline.

The advanced study program of the Center for Advanced Engineering Study, through the help of the appropriate M.I.T. faculty, offers each participant an individual program tailored to his own background, needs and objectives and allows him to draw upon any of the resources of M.I.T. for which he is qualified. These resources include the special subjects and seminars offered by the center, regular graduate and undergraduate subjects, seminars offered by the departments and interdisciplinary centers, and the laboratories, libraries, and other facilities.

The center also offers a full-time study program in systematic analysis, in which a complete program has been developed for a group selected from a number of federal government agencies. The subjects are specially designed for, and limited to, the participants in the program.

The experience gained in offering full-time study programs is useful in developing the most meaningful programs for professional self-study. After teaching the material to one or more groups in the full-time study program, the instructors know the best way to approach the subject for a self-study format. They know which aspects of the subject are most difficult and, therefore, require more detailed information. They know what questions to expect and how to answer them and what study problems and outside readings are most beneficial.

The experience gained in developing and offering the advanced study program and the systematic analysis program would also be of great value in developing full-time programs for physicians and medically-oriented engineers.

The special subjects developed in a full-time study program for physicians and biomedical engineers could be "packaged," as described above, for use by others engaged in teaching and research who could not spend one or more academic terms at M.I.T. and Harvard.

In conjunction with Harvard Medical School, a full-time study program for physicians and medical researchers operating within the framework of the Center for Advanced Engineering Study could accommodate one or more of the following types of men.

A. Professors in medical schools would spend their time learning more about the engineering and the physical sciences relevant to their teaching and research. They would also attend seminars and conferences concerned with the latest medical advances. By having this opportunity to update their knowledge, they could improve their teaching and have a favorable influence on their students.

B. Younger physicians, just finishing their residencies, would spend a year in full-time study learning the physics, mathematics, and engineering they need to pursue fruitful careers in academic medicine or research in the life sciences. The program would include research involvement.

C. Engineers and physical scientists, in order to use their knowledge effectively in the field of biomedical engineering, must have a good understanding of the life sciences. The subjects they would need would depend on their interests. The program should be flexible enough to accommodate different interests, and it should also include laboratory research opportunities. However, there could be a "core" set of subjects specially developed for them, possibly consisting of biochemistry, physiology, neurophysiology, pathology, and anatomy.

D. Established researchers with formal backgrounds in medicine would benefit from learning more about engineering principles and the physical sciences.

The full-time study programs would be nondegree, continuing education programs intended for mature, highly motivated individuals who already have professional credentials, either an M.D. degree or an advanced degree in engineering or science.

If a program for a few teachers or researchers were implemented within the framework of the M.I.T. Center for Advanced Engineering Study, an individual program would be arranged for each participant drawing on the resources of M.I.T. and Harvard. In some subject areas, special tutors or guided self-study would be arranged.

If a program were implemented for fifteen men with similar backgrounds and objectives, special subjects could be developed tailored to the needs of the group. In this case, participants would attend their classes together, and the classes would be restricted to the members of the program. In some areas, special offerings are preferable to attending regular classes offered for less experienced, younger (but from a prerequisite point of view, often better prepared) undergraduate and graduate students.

The problems with the full-time study program are primarily funding and staffing. Funding would provide each participant with a stipend roughly equivalent to his previous year's income, pay moving expenses for him and his family to come to the Boston area, and pay the educational costs. The educational cost can be estimated at about $5,000 per academic year per participant, plus several hundred dollars for each participant for books and supplies.

If special subjects are offered, interested faculty must be found who are willing to participate and who can be relieved of a large portion of their regular teaching duties. Senior faculty members of both M.I.T. and Harvard not otherwise involved in the program must be willing to give informal seminars on the latest developments in their fields. Providing research and guided self-study opportunities for the participants also requires staff.

Staffing is not so serious a problem if the participants attend regular graduate and undergraduate subjects at M.I.T. and Harvard. It is important, however, to provide contacts with faculty who have interests similar to those of the participants. It is also important for each participant to arrange a study program that matches the scholarly activities of Harvard and M.I.T. with his needs.

The participants also require adequate study and relaxation facilities. It is not sufficient to enroll these men the way regular students are enrolled. The men need private studies; they need a lounge in which to hold informal discussions; and they need to have planned activities that bring them together as a group. The Center for Advanced Engineering Study has these facilities and activities for the participants in the programs it now offers. The center, in cooperation with Harvard Medical School and those at M.I.T. involved in medical research and biomedical engineering, could offer similar facilities and activities for continued education programs in medicine and biomedical engineering.

A final problem in offering the full-time study program for men with medical backgrounds is that this background is usually weak in mathematics and physics. Therefore, even for men who pursue programs made up of regular subject offerings, special review mathematics and physics subjects should probably be developed for the summer preceding the first regular academic term. These review subjects should be related to the life sciences in some meaningful way.

Task Group Report on Diagnostic Instrumentation

Stephen K. Burns
ASSISTANT PROFESSOR IN ELECTRICAL ENGINEERING
MASSACHUSETTS INSTITUTE OF TECHNOLOGY, CHAIRMAN

Saul Aronow
ASSOCIATE APPLIED PHYSICIST
MEDICAL ENGINEERING LABORATORY
MASSACHUSETTS GENERAL HOSPITAL

George B. Benedek
PROFESSOR OF PHYSICS
MASSACHUSETTS INSTITUTE OF TECHNOLOGY

Alastair W. B. Cunningham
ASSOCIATE IN PATHOLOGY
PETER BENT BRIGHAM HOSPITAL

Melvin H. Rodman
ASSOCIATE MEDICAL DIRECTOR
MEDICAL DEPARTMENT
MASSACHUSETTS INSTITUTE OF TECHNOLOGY

William A. Simon
RESEARCH ASSOCIATE IN PHYSIOLOGY
HARVARD MEDICAL SCHOOL

Warren E. C. Wacker
ASSISTANT PROFESSOR IN MEDICINE
PETER BENT BRIGHAM HOSPITAL

This report is concerned with the development of specific techniques and devices relevant to experimental studies in the life and health sciences and the development and improvement of instrumentation for use in clinical screening and diagnosis. The problem is dealt with in two parts: first, the characteristics of an adequate diagnostic test are discussed and specific examples are offered; second, problems concerning the handling of large quantities of data obtained by diagnostic instrumentation are considered.

The ideal diagnostic test would be noninvasive and nontraumatic; it would produce its results instantaneously and in the appropriate form for those using the information; it would provide for a permanent and easily accessible record of its results; and finally it would be better and less costly than present tests. Admittedly this is an ideal projection, but it is an ideal sufficiently realistic to provide useful guidelines for developing new systems and modifying old ones.

The physician presently employs a number of noninvasive diagnostic techniques. He palpates for abnormal deep structures; he auscultates for noises and excites resonances by percussing the body surfaces; he peers into body orifices; and he feels for abnormally warm areas. Roentgenograms allow him to examine outlines of deep structures. But the availability of new techniques suggest that much more can probably be done. Not only can present methods be improved but new methods based on recently developed techniques of physical measurements can be developed. For example, other physical probes—such as acoustic, magnetic, or electric fields—might be applied to visualize internal structure. Molecular or nuclear resonance phenomena could be exploited in like manner. Indeed, there are many physical phenomena that have not yet been used to examine structure and activity within the body, and these should be examined for such applicability.

The use of such phenomena to provide measurements equivalent to presently used tests might mean that the necessary amount of sample material or degree of patient exposure could be substantially reduced. Materials now assayed by chemical tests might be estimated by some other means, such as nuclear magnetic resonance. For such substances as serum or cerebralspinal fluid, this could mean a significant decrease in discomfort or inconvenience to the patient. Image-enhancement procedures, so successfully applied in modern astronomy to examine other planets, could be used to improve the quality of the X-ray images available to the clinician.

The idea is to innovate rather than to try and improve upon the tests that are now used. New measurements are continually evolving, and we should be concerned with their potential medical applications.

The following suggestions illustrate some new techniques that hold promise for the field of opthalmology. Roughly speaking, the major diseases of the eye can be divided into the following three general categories: (1) glaucoma, (2) retinal detachment, and (3) opacification (cataract and corneal edema). Each could benefit substantially from improvements in diagnostic instrumentation of the kind outlined below.

1. *Glaucoma:* Glaucoma results from reduction of the flow of aqueous from the anterior chamber through Schlemm's canal into the blood vessels of the sclera. This reduction, combined with the regular increase of aqueous produced by the ciliary body, results in raised intraocular pressure, which is transmitted to the base of the optic nerve. The pressure on the optic nerve base produces first a deformity of the nerve fibers, then a reduction in visual field, leading finally to blindness. There are thirty to forty thousand people each year who lose their sight because of glaucoma.

Early and reliable diagnosis is vital to the effective treatment of glaucoma. Present methods of diagnosis involve measuring intraocular pressure and the resistance of aqueous flow out of the eye (tonography). These methods are difficult and subject to systematic error; simple, more accurate ones are needed. One possible approach is to first apply a fluctuating stress to the sclera, then measure the resulting strain on the sclera as a function of the frequency of the stress. The amplitude and phase relationship between stress and strain should permit a measurement of the flow rate out of the eye.

2. *Retinal Detachment:* For reasons that are not yet understood, the vitreous sometimes shrinks away from the choroid and the retina. This can lead to detachment of the retina from the choroid and consequent blindness.

Again diagnosis in the form of a clear visualization of the retina and the vitreous is very important. Present instruments, which examine the retina through the cornea, have a narrow view angle. A highly skilled physician is required to conduct the examination, and even under the best conditions the doctor would like to see much more than the instruments now permit.

One very promising area for progress here is the use of the low-power laser as illumination; this entails photographing the image of the retina as a hologram. The development of such a technique would allow the opthalmologist to make a three-dimensional examination of the morphology of the detached retina at a whole range of angles and with no time limit. Were this successful, it would profoundly affect the technique of diagnosis of retinal detachment.

3. *Opacification:* A problem should not, of course, be considered unworthy of attention because it does not involve radically new application of technology. The slit-lamp microscope is highly useful; though it could be even more so if it yielded quantitative information. It is presently the most effective single instrument used in the diagnosis of eye disease. However, in these instruments, as conventionally designed, there are no facilities for the quantitative measurement of the turbidity or scattering from the cornea and lens.

The slit-lamp microscope could be adapted to include photoelectric detection devices that would permit quantitative detection of early cataract and corneal edema. Such an instrument would also be useful in the proper fitting of contact lenses, since the points of incorrect fit generally show clouding of the cornea. A precise detection for such clouding would be of great utility for optometrists, and early quantitative measurement of corneal edema and cataract would also be valuable to clinicians.

The ability to measure rapidly and easily the distribution of blood or other substances either for a specific region, a specific system, or the organism as a whole is of enormous significance for work in the three major disabling diseases—heart disease, cancer, and stroke. This problem could fit rather well into the academic research environment: there is a specific focus or goal; yet there are a number of possible approaches, some involving fundamental research.

Included in this would be the development of a simple nontraumatic system for estimating pulmonary function, including regional mechanical properties, ventilation, and perfusion of the lung. A reliable means for estimating the distribution and dynamics of both gases and blood in the chest is also urgently needed. The possibility of tagging cells in the circulatory system magnetically and observing their dynamic behaviour or the development of an instrument to provide rapid imaging of internal radioisotopic tracer distribution may be steps in this direction. For the latter application, good resolution (3 millimeters) at high speed (0.1 seconds per frame) is desired to do two-dimensional dynamic studies. Initially, of course, this requires fundamental physics and image-processing developments. Visualization of the results is a critical area of the problem.

A noninvasive method for estimating total cardiac output would also be of great significance. Such an instrument would be invaluable for evaluating drug efficacy in the treatment of congestive heart failure, as well as have a possible predictive value in treating other circulatory diseases. Present systems of estimating cardiac output involve catheters and arterial punctures and are at best an unpleasant experience for the patient. Perhaps ultrasonic Doppler sounders or a very sensitive magnetic flow measuring apparatus combined with statistical methods might be applied to this problem; or new approaches to the phonocardiogram (Apex cardiogram), or ballistocardiogram might prove useful. Such a development program, of course, would involve close collaboration between physiologists and communications engineers.

Another item that would require considerable cooperation and collaboration between engineering and medical groups, one that is of considerable practical significance at the present time, involves the development of a simple, inexpensive method for detecting, analyzing, and displaying premature ventricular contractions that could be used with a large population. This might be done either in a coronary intensive care unit, or be put into general portable use with ambulatory patients. Such an ectopic beat detector should be small, easily portable, not prohibitively expensive, and capable of characterizing normal and abnormal cardiac activity in an electrocardiogram. Thus, normal cardiac events might be characterized by pulse output while abnormal cardiac output might be immediately classified according to the nature of the abnormality; or a means might be provided for the data to be recorded or transmitted to a device capable of such classification. This device would be of tremendous importance in treating cardiovascular disease characterized by transient arrythmias or ectopic beats. It might be of even greater importance to the field of preventive medicine in predicting electrical catastrophes of the cardiovascular system.

At the present time such an application is difficult to evaluate because of the enormous amount of data to be analyzed. The information rate of several thousand bits per second required to represent the electrocardiographic waveform might possibly be reduced by some preprocessing, to make extensive monitoring of screening programs more feasible. Although there is little published work in this area, there is considerable interest being shown by the medical electronics industry, biomedical engineering facilities in some schools, and clinicians themselves. Needless to say, close cooperation between physician and engineer is required for the successful evaluation of such a system.

The vast amount of data obtained by modern diagnostic methods demands that new and more efficient means of handling this material be developed. For example, characterization of cardiovascular activity over long intervals is needed. Virtually all analysis of electrocardiographic activity is presently based upon visual inspection of electrocardiograms, i.e., a time series recorded on paper. Because this gives hours and days of data rather than seconds and minutes, such a system makes it difficult to summarize and display electrocardiographic information. Therefore, new formats are indicated. For example, a summary might be "Rate varied from 62.5 to 151 beats per minute. 242 ectopic events of similar morphology," and so on. or it might be a visual display that allows both trends and individual transient events to be observed. Again, close collaboration with the physician is required since the characterization must be useful in forming clinical evaluations.

In contrast, the sort of project which would require minimal collaboration with physicians might be the development of a device to provide fast, easy spectral analysis of the electroencephalogram. Such analysis may be used as one criterion for clinical death or for monitoring anaesthesia during surgery. Since the spectral characteristics of the electroencephalogram are most often referred to by a neurologist examining a record, such a spectral analyzer could be of considerable utility. Although many such analyzers have been built, only recently have developments in electronics allowed economical construction.

Another approach to the data proliferation problem that has received considerable attention lately is the proposal for the establishment of a comprehensive, automated clinical laboratory. Not only would such a laboratory be of value to the individual patient but it would also permit meaningful observations to be made concerning the distribution of physiological variables in a large population. Sequential observations of a relatively stable population over the course of several years would provide valuable information for time studies of health and disease, and base-line data is essential for any automated analysis and evaluation of clinical material.

In some instances the laboratory could replace the physician; for example, in preemployment screening, annual examination of workers in hazardous occupations, and voluntary periodical health surveys of employees. In other words it could serve as an efficient auxiliary to the physician. Furthermore, since the data would be stored and retrieved by computer, the information developed could be used easily and efficiently for research and educational purposes. In other instances screening could aid the physician, for example, the screening of a symptomatic population.

Improvements in data handling in clinical laboratories concerned with highly specific problems are also possible. Automatic enzyme screenings, for example, in the detection of PKU (phenylketonuria), could perhaps be handled in a single regional center serving a number of hospitals. More general improvements in laboratory procedures are also called for; a fool-proof method of identifying laboratory samples would be an enormous help in relieving the terrible burden of bookkeeping which occupies the bulk of the present unsatisfactory clinical laboratory efforts. Record processing, distribution, and storage is a major problem today. An *integrated* system for information processing is vital and should receive very high priority. What is required is a unique method of associating a particular sample with a particular patient. This means that a mode of identification must be readable by both human observers and by machines. It is possible that a coded additive could be introduced to each sample and hence automatically analyzed along with the sample itself. Alternatives include a machine-readable paper label or a uniquely identifiable bottle or container for the sample.

Industry and Diagnostic Instrumentation

Industry has taken very considerable notice of medical electronics. A recent issue of *Medical Electronic News* contained advertisements from 113 different companies. There are at least five journals published specifically about bioengineering. All of the major aerospace concerns have groups working in "bioengineering." Economists predict that the defense dollar will eventually be channeled into other problems of society and a large portion to the area of health care. The principal computer manufacturers are all involved in medical care systems associated with their computer products. Industry represents a very considerable potential and should be considered quite carefully to avoid paralleling its efforts.

Industry has demonstrated itself capable of producing an instrument very quickly after the technical specifications and the need have been established. For example, the flame photometer was in use in the clinical chemistry lab in less than five years after the publication of the suggestive basic research. Transistorized averaging computers were on the market three years after the first transistorized computer was built in the laboratory. Delimiting problems and establishing appropriate specifications seems to be the principle difficulty faced by industry in applying today's technology to problems in medicine.

There are several criticisms of the medical electronics industry that have repeatedly been voiced. One is the lack of the "systems" approach. Manufacturers want to be involved in a tightly defined product area. They want their product to be independent of outside apparatus. Rarely are manufacturers cooperative about interconnecting their apparatus with the apparatus of another. They regard their data and their design as proprietary and are reluctant to communicate it. Automated record keeping and process control demands a measurement *system* rather than a collection of instruments.

Another criticism is that human engineering fails to accompany many devices and tests now on the market. The apparatus sold to the clinical laboratory is often a duplicate of one developed by a research worker. It requires skilled operation and interpretation and often produces more information than is desired. Instruments must be designed to be operated easier and to require less calibration and adjustment.

It is difficult for industry to adequately evaluate the efficacy of a new or different technique and hence difficult to get the development accepted and marketed. Frequently the design engineering is inadequate, for once a company has committed itself to manufacturing a particular piece of apparatus there are few changes made. The design of an instrument or a measurement system for clinical application should be a continual interaction between engineers and physicians. The engineer should have some idea of the physician's problems; and conversely the physician must realize some of the possibilities and limitations of engineering. One good way of doing this is by working together.

The committee agreed that there is need for an intermediary between the physician who uses an instrument and the industry that produces it. But there is considerable debate as to whether such a "service" facility could fit into the M.I.T. attitude toward engineering and the Harvard attitude about medicine, both of which favor research over application in the belief that a coherent research program can be more visible and more easily evaluated than a series of unrelated efforts such as often characterizes applied engineering or medicine.

Although problems exist, members of the committee do not seem to be particularly dissatisfied with the ad hoc nature of the present interactions between engineering and medicine at M.I.T. and Harvard. The problem areas considered were those of funding, professional recognition, and students.

Most joint projects are funded by means of a research grant to a specific group for a specific problem. These can usually withstand a certain amount of borrowing to seed new research projects, but extensive "fishing" is not possible. Often joint projects are not pure enough to be considered solid and are difficult to fund by research grants.

Professional recognition seemed to be of considerable concern, particularly among committee members who have achieved such recognition. It was pointed out that it would be extremely difficult for a junior faculty member in the physics department to conduct a program of research in the diseases of the eye and still remain in the physics department: it might be good research but it isn't physics. There are similar problems in attracting young M.D.s who are trying to establish a professional reputation.

The committee was concerned with this question of institutional form. From the discussion, several general requirements were developed: (1) there must be a place for people to talk; (2) as a part of a university it must be concerned with training people; and (3) it must have full academic status and provide a first-class professional opportunity.

Several specific forms were discussed. These were (1) The present system in which individuals, laboratories and departments are funded so that interested faculty receive grants from the Department of Defense, the National Science Foundation, the National Institutes of Health, and so on. This arrangement was felt to be acceptable for senior faculty but not for junior faculty whose tenure considerations had to be taken into account. (2) Establishment of a loosely organized laboratory like Research Laboratory of Electronics which does some central fund raising and provides some support services but leaves direction of research to the individual worker. This structure had considerable appeal; it is easy to initiate new or different research in such an environment. (Large-scale goal-directed projects are somewhat less appealing because such extensive support is required.) Such an institutional form avoids the issue of faculty and professional status. (3) This, in turn, suggested that an Instrumentation-Lincoln Laboratory sort of facility be established with an extensive support facility. This structure did not generate much enthusiasm among the committee members. Very large projects might be better handled by an organization like N.I.H. (4) An academic department with a strong committment to instrumentation could be established and would be able to provide support and facilities. This department would be empowered to make faculty appointments at M.I.T. and Harvard, deal with students, and administer research. This form held considerable appeal for the majority of the members of the committee because of its teaching function. It was pointed out that a university should not be involved in doing something that could be accomplished at Massachusetts General Hospital or Arthur D. Little, Inc. (5) Considerable thought was given to opportunities offered by an ambulatory care center to serve the Cambridge community; it would be formally affiliated with both Harvard and M.I.T. and have the status of an academic department. This center would have many of the facilities of a general hospital but would allow for engineering and teaching functions on the premises. It would allow research into such problems as how medical care can best be delivered in terms of sociology and economics, as well as medicine and engineering. Most members of the committee felt that such an ambulatory care center would fill their personal requirements. (6) Establishing a new general hospital was considered unsuitable. It involves a very long term committment and is highly goal orientated. It would have to be staffed with presently available people and use accepted diagnostic techniques. Its ongoing function could not be interrupted for the sake of research.

Task Group Report on Diagnostic Processes

William B. Kannel
CLINICAL ASSOCIATE IN PREVENTIVE MEDICINE AT
HARVARD MEDICAL SCHOOL
HEART DISEASE EPIDEMIOLOGICAL STUDY
U.S. PUBLIC HEALTH SERVICE IN FRAMINGHAM, CHAIRMAN

Osler L. Peterson
VISITING PROFESSOR OF PREVENTIVE MEDICINE
MEMBER OF THE FACULTY OF PUBLIC ADMINISTRATION
HARVARD MEDICAL SCHOOL

Rhett Tsao
CAMBRIDGE SCIENTIFIC CENTER
IBM CORPORATION

The report centers on the determination of how the unique range of skills, resources, and personnel of Harvard and the Massachusetts Institute of Technology, working in close, integrated collaboration, can be brought to bear on the process of diagnosis with the aim of achieving more accurate, precise, and efficient diagnosis of existing illness or unusual vulnerability to disease.

More specifically, these objectives entail an examination of the following:

1. To explore the nature of the diagnostic process and discover whether or not it is a uniform, standard process.
2. To determine the deficiencies in contemporary diagnostic practices.
3. To establish how an organized multidisciplinary team might explore and improve clinical diagnosis.
4. To specify what skills should comprise such a team.
5. To explore the relevant technological advances in medicine, mathematics, biostatistics, nosology, machine data processing, information storage and retrieval, automated laboratory procedures, physiological monitoring, diagnostic instrumentation, and biomedical engineering that might be applied to the problem.
6. To identify specific departments, groups, and individuals working in these or related areas who might be available to collaborate in an attack on the problem.

Specific Objectives Worthy of Consideration

1. To explore the role of computers and high-speed data processing techniques in medical diagnosis. Possible roles include: (1) substitution for the physician in history taking and analysis of diagnostic information; (2) use as a laboratory tool to assist the physician in making a differential diagnosis; (3) an aid to the study of the diagnostic process; (4) a means for storage and rapid retrieval of cumulative information concerning characteristic, cardinal findings useful in diagnosis; (5) to explore methods of classifying disease which may be more helpful for differential diagnosis; (6) a teaching device for learning differential diagnosis.

2. To institute a reexamination of the methodology

and concepts employed in the diagnostic process by a multidisciplinary team in order to define the nature of the problem, its logical structure, and the actual set of processes the physician employs in arriving at a diagnosis, and to then examine alternative methodologies and formal equivalences and concepts to arrive at an improved diagnostic process. This would entail an examination of the process of diagnosis as a problem in pattern recognition and a reexamination of the basic assumptions behind the method of classification now employed for medical diagnosis. New and more useful labels for disease should be sought. An analysis should be made of techniques that lead to a high rate of correct diagnosis in contrast with those that lead to frequent failures.

3. To apply more sophisticated analytical techniques to help distinguish between diseases that share cardinal manifestations. Techniques that could be explored include discriminant function analysis, stepwise regression analysis, factor analysis, decision analysis, Bayes' Theorem, mathematical linguistics, and theory of algorithms, among others.

4. To apply the skills of electrical engineers, physicians, computer experts, and biostatisticians to the tasks of devising improvements in the various aspects of the diagnostic process, such as history taking, complete and rapid retrieval of past history of medical findings, and the synthesis of these findings into a diagnosis. To this core group additional skills available in each institution could be added when required to meet specific needs.

Automatic coding (precoded) forms for obtaining medical information should be developed. These are essential for automatic data processing. These should be designed for use in inpatient and outpatient institutions in the Harvard complex.

5. To explore means for devising a computerized reference and consultative diagnostic service that is easily accessible, rapid, and kept up to date. Information should be made available concerning tests useful in establishing the diagnosis of a given disease entity: the range of normal values; diagnostic work-up appropriate for a given set of complaints; how to carry out complex diagnostic procedures; where uncommon diagnostic tests

may be obtained; consultative service for interpretation of ECG, X-rays, and laboratory findings. As new, sophisticated, highly specialized techniques become available, the physician must immediately be made aware of their availability and the way to interpret the findings.

6. Develop diagnostic procedures and techniques appropriate for periodic health examinations designed to detect asymptomatic persons vulnerable to though not yet afflicted with the major health hazards (coronary disease, emphysema, diabetes, and so forth). This would be especially applicable to the usually undetected diseases that can be controlled. Knowledge concerning the detection and prophylactic management of the premorbid state is in a nearly primitive stage. Well-designed, prospective epidemiological studies are needed to provide further information on the early detection of vulnerable persons, factors of risk, and early asymptomatic disease. It should be possible to use, for epidemiological research, the health records of students, faculty, and alumni of the two institutions, as well as outpatient department records in the various hospitals in order to obtain information on the natural history of disease.

Specific Proposals for Action Programs

The objectives of these would be to implement stated goals.

1. A model diagnostic clinic. This would be a demonstration project designed by engineers, business administrators, biostatisticians, and physicians for the purpose of operating a diagnostic subspecialty clinic. A cardiac clinic is recommended as a good choice since this is an important problem and many sophisticated diagnostic modalities are available to evaluate.

The chief objectives would be: (1) to modify existing diagnostic tests to make them more reliable and more valid, and less expensive, traumatic, hazardous, and unpleasant; (2) to devise new tests employing engineering technology available to evaluate cardiac function, heart murmurs, heart chamber enlargement; (3) to study and improve the process of collecting and analyzing data for diagnosis; (4) to study the decision process in getting the patient from complaint to definitive therapy; (5) to determine the amount and nature of the input necessary, desirable, essential, and optimal for making accurate differential diagnoses—this should be determined for each of the major disease constellations in cardiology; (6) to devise, employ, and test out new equipment for improving physical diagnosis in cardiology; (7) to devise precoded standard forms for uniformity in obtaining a more comprehensive appraisal and to allow and facilitate data processing.

This would be used to explore the utility and feasibility of setting up in each subspecialty, in the various hospital outpatient department clinics, specifically designed units for the diagnosis of referred ambulatory patients. Such units should employ the most advanced technology in automated laboratory techniques, for example, biomedical aids to physical diagnosis, and advanced radiographic techniques. This could provide a workshop for exploration and evaluation of innovations in diagnosis of disease.

2. A study project designed to investigate and analyze currently employed diagnostic techniques in one of the Harvard-affiliated outpatient clinics. Techniques that have had high rates of correct diagnoses should be sought out, and those that lead to frequent failures should be identified. A reexamination of the methodology and concepts employed in the diagnostic process should be undertaken by a multidisciplinary team in order to define the nature of the process, its logical structure, and the actual set of processes that practicing physicians employ in arriving at a diagnosis.

For each of the major disciplines (such as surgery, orthopedics, cardiology, gastroenterology, and hematology) the sequential process of elimination and ordering of possibilities, the minimal criteria acceptable for identifying a disease with reasonable specificity, and the amount and nature of the input desirable, essential, and optimal for differential diagnosis should be determined for each of the major disease constellations in each subspecialty.

3. The collective experience of physicians is an untapped source of data related to the diagnostic process. With the use of automatic data processing equipment, it should be possible to collect, store, and analyze such material as can be obtained from all the major teaching institutions in the Harvard complex. A central computer

memory bank could be developed to store, to process, and to analyze diagnostic information, continuously and automatically, accumulated from the major diagnostic centers. This should provide a constant revision of probability estimates of particular disease entities that will account for a given constellation of findings and the range of diseases which must be included in the differential diagnosis. This should improve information concerning the cardinal characteristics unique to a particular disease.

The major obstacles to accomplishing this are the lack of a proper framework for the use of this collective experience, uncertainty concerning what data to collect and store, and how to ascertain the quality of the input.

4. Development of a computerized device to be employed as an aid in teaching diagnosis at Harvard.

5. Development of a computerized diagnostic reference and consultative service. This should be readily and immediately accessible by telephone. Answers should be given over the phone on standby service, to be followed the next day by a mailed printout. Information such as: diseases to consider and appropriate tests to run, additional information required to narrow differential diagnosis, where to obtain diagnostic tests, range of normal values and diagnostic levels of "abnormality" for tests, methods of carrying out diagnostic procedures, diagnostic work-up appropriate, and informative up-to-date references on diagnosis of specific disease entities. Such a service could be developed first for hospital personnel in the Harvard complex before more general application is attempted.

6. Development of an automated multitest screening laboratory. There should be established a screening clinic to detect asymptomatic disease and abnormalities indicating vulnerability to the major contemporary health hazards among the Harvard employee, student, and faculty health units. A multiphasic screening procedure should be designed to detect persons vulnerable to coronary heart disease, stroke, diabetes, hypertension, early glaucoma, and emphysema, among others.

This prophylactic screening should be tied in with a mobile medical establishment to follow through and implement an effective prophylactic program designed to delay the onset of symptomatic disease.

Physicians are too scarce to be employed in examining asymptomatic populations. Health screening clinics must employ a sufficiently sensitive and specific series of tests that can be administered by nonprofessional personnel and analyzed by automated techniques. These should be developed by a multidisciplinary team.

7. Emergency room diagnostic clinic. This is an environment that demands prompt, accurate, efficient diagnostic procedures, critical decisions, and immediate effective therapy. Disposition as to admission to the hospital or return to home must be made.

There is a growing demand by the public for emergency room services. Physicians now tend to evaluate serious problems there rather than at home or in their offices. The emergency room is the point of the greatest contact between hospital and public. (In the past ten years, the number of emergency room visits has at least tripled in most institutions.) This warrants an emergency room chief and staff and first-rate diagnostic facilities to expedite handling of these immediate, often life-threatening problems.

It is recommended that a team of physicians, engineers, systems analysts, and the like, make a study, then plan and implement an ideal or model emergency room diagnostic unit to aid in achieving a rapid and accurate appraisal of emergency room patients.

The emergency room is a place were a rapid, accurate diagnosis, treatment, and disposition is imperative. The outcome is usually dramatically obvious in a relatively short time and appears to be a good place to study innovations designed to improve the efficiency and precision of diagnosis.

Some General Considerations

The problems currently encountered in the diagnostic process should be identified in order both to determine the state-of-the-art available and to identify needs. To assist in this, a comprehensive and systematic review of the literature dealing with the process of diagnosis should be made.

Some of the deficiencies in diagnostic practice are obvious, including: false or inadequate information; faulty or incomplete physical findings; improper synthesis of diagnostic information; and failure to consider all possibilities. It seems reasonable to proceed on the assumption that an improvement in each of these parameters would also improve the diagnostic process.

Diagnosis may be defined as the art, science, or act of recognizing disease or a pathologic state from signs, symptoms, or laboratory data, taking into account the course of illness, response to specific therapy, and even the outcomes.

For an examination of alternative approaches, this needs to be translated into mathematical models. The ingredients of a diagnosis include the following interdigitating and overlapping components: (1) time-connected constellations of weighted manifestations of complaints, physical findings and laboratory results that may be of localizing value or indicative of a general nonspecific response of the organism; (2) minimal criteria for disease based on the weighted groups of manifestations; (3) a consideration of all admissable reasonable hypotheses; (4) a judgment based on a knowledge of etiology, pathology, and physiology, as well as empirical correlations.

Classically, the process begins with a chief complaint and present illness, essentially a data-collection process including a check for internal consistency. Analysis of data is carried on simultaneously with the formulation of tentative hypotheses serving as guides to the collection of more data. A formulative state then ensues utilizing a fund of medical knowledge, experience, and insight. This is further elaborated and rechecked by reentering the data-collection phase. To ascertain that no important item has been missed, a system review is undertaken to check for cardinal signs and symptoms of deranged organ function. By means of classification schemes and diagnostic trees, a tentative diagnosis or clinical impression is reached. Finally, a diagnostic formulation is reached in terms of implications for care, management, prognosis, disposition, prophylaxis, and even employability and insurability. This may lead to therapy before a definitive diagnosis is reached by eliciting pathognomonic findings through laboratory or other diagnostic tests. The response to such therapy, or lack of it, may also contribute to the diagnostic process and indicate a need for reentry into the data-collection phase.

This is indeed a complex process with many pitfalls. There are only a limited number of ways in which an organism can react to noxious stimuli. Consequently, there must be considerable overlap of symptoms and signs for a variety of etiologically distinct "diseases." A poisoning, a neoplasm, an infection, a metabolic failure, a vascular occlusion may all produce an identical constellation of symptoms and signs. It is also common, especially in advanced age, for a number of diseases to coexist in the same individual.

The course of the disease, response to specific therapy, and, fortunately, certain pathognomonic biochemical and physiologic findings often allow a distinction among these. The trick is to know when to make the appropriate pathognomonic test, as the test may be costly, unpleasant, hazardous, and difficult to obtain.

Furthermore, various types of diagnoses are distinguished: (1) etiologic (e.g., shock due to myocardial infarction); (2) physiologic (e.g., hypertension, hypovolemia, anoxia, anuria, diminished cardiac output); (3) biochemical (e.g., acidosis, hypoxia, ketosis); or (4) merely a syndrome of unknown etiology.

Types of diagnoses are also classified according to the kinds of evidence used in arriving at them. Thus, there are anatomic, pathologic, physical, and laboratory diagnoses, for example. Differential diagnosis is the label for the process of distinguishing among different diseases that resemble each other. Clinical diagnosis implies diagnosis by means of techniques readily available to the clinician rather than the pathologist.

At the very least the "diagnosis" must assign a name to a "disease" or constellation of findings. Often, but not always, it connotes knowledge of causal factors. It implies that its character has been determined as to type with some estimate of the severity and kind of damage and should forecast the probable course and duration of the morbid process.

Diagnosis may be divided into groups: well-defined entities with clear etiologies and at the other extreme those that are entirely descriptive and of unknown etiologies. The criteria employed in establishing a diagnosis may involve primarily gross anatomical defects, microscopic anatomical changes, specific etiologic agents, specific deficiencies, genetic aberrations, physiologic or biochemical abnormalities, constellations of clinical symptoms and signs, organ system involvement, or simply a description of abnormalities.

Some diseases are diagnosed principally by a history of complaints (angina, claudication), others entirely on physical findings (pterygium, psoriasis), and still others by biochemical findings (adult onset diabetes).

The foregoing indicates certain difficulties in coping with the process of diagnosis, including the absence of a unified concept of "disease," the lack of universally accepted definitions for diseases, the fact that not all diseases are discrete and clearly distinguishable from one another, that there is no fixed number of diseases, and that definitions of disease are continually changing.

There is no need to illustrate and detail the formal procedure for obtaining and processing data for making diagnostic decisions. This involves determining the likelihood of probable diseases for a given constellation of symptoms and signs, the amount of information likely to be gained from further testing, the possibility of untoward side effects from the tests and the value and utility of the outcomes that might accrue from alternative courses of action. Maximizing the probability of a cure must be balanced against side effects (including death) and dollar costs.

The modern emphasis in diagnosis is justifiably on early diagnosis: the interpretation of minimal subjective symptoms and seemingly trivial signs. More use needs to be made of therapeutic tests as legitimate adjutants to diagnostic information. Changes in body chemistry and metabolism that may permit recognition and treatment of functional disturbances before irreversible organic damage has occurred should be sought out.

While the classical sequence of first obtaining history information, then physical findings, and finally selected laboratory tests may justifiably be questioned, there is much to recommend it. However obtaining certain routine biochemical and physiologic information on every patient, regardless of his complaints, is also easily justified. This is especially relevant if a premorbid vulnerable state is to be detected in its asymptomatic phase.

Thus, a battery of biochemical tests including blood urea nitrogen, blood sugar, uric acid, hemoglobin, cholesterol, and possibly certain other biochemical determinations can be recommended periodically for everyone, as can an electrocardiogram, chest X-ray, blood pressure determination, body weight check, vital capacity measurement, expiratory flow rate, and an intraocular tension measurement.

Emphasis in all these endeavors should be placed on conditions that respond to treatment or those that may be prevented by timely intervention, rather than on rare, bizarre, often terminal, clinical curiosities.

Task Group Report on Image Processing and Visualization Techniques

Oleh J. Tretiak
LECTURER IN ELECTRICAL ENGINEERING
MASSACHUSETTS INSTITUTE OF TECHNOLOGY, CHAIRMAN

John F. Burke
ASSOCIATE VISITING SURGEON
MASSACHUSETTS GENERAL HOSPITAL

Paul R. Gross
PROFESSOR OF BIOLOGY
MASSACHUSETTS INSTITUTE OF TECHNOLOGY

Thomas S. Huang
ASSOCIATE PROFESSOR OF ELECTRICAL ENGINEERING
MASSACHUSETTS INSTITUTE OF TECHNOLOGY

Edward Kaplan
COMPUTING CENTER
HARVARD UNIVERSITY

Lawrence Razavi
BOSTON CITY HOSPITAL

William F. Schreiber
ASSOCIATE PROFESSOR OF ELECTRICAL ENGINEERING
MASSACHUSETTS INSTITUTE OF TECHNOLOGY

Charles L. Seitz III
INSTRUCTOR IN ELECTRICAL ENGINEERING
MASSACHUSETTS INSTITUTE OF TECHNOLOGY

Edward W. Webster
PHYSICIST, RADIOLOGY
MASSACHUSETTS GENERAL HOSPITAL

Collaborative efforts among biologists and engineers to apply existing techniques to the handling of visual data and to develop new techniques for this purpose are underway in a number of laboratories in the M.I.T.-Harvard complex and elsewhere. Much of this work involves fundamental research on basic engineering methods required to manipulate visual information efficiently and effectively. While emphasis is thus on methodology, the extremely wide range of practical applications evident in both the projected and ongoing projects detailed below indicates the enormous potential inherent in this area of research.

This potential is well illustrated by the current work in computer photometry. This is a technique to measure accurately the composition and mass of cellular and subcellular constituents by using a combination of manual and computer methods. An appropriately stained sample is scanned, and the data are transmitted into the computer. Using a graphic input device, the experimenter then delineates the perimeter of the stained images, and after applying suitable correction factors, the computer calculates the total mass (or some other desired parameter). It is hoped that refinements of this technique can be used to perform karyotypes or collect data to test karyotype algorithms.

In a related use of the computer, efforts are now under way to study the morphology of Golgi-stained neurons with an on-line system consisting of a camera-lucida, a graphic input device, and a means of measuring the focus control position on a microscope. The data collected through this system could be used either to draw these neurons in an arbitrary orientation or as input to some program that might classify the neurons. Such projects demand development of new and more efficient ways of storing three-dimensional shapes on a computer.

Application of such techniques to the teaching of anatomy is an interesting possibility. Information regarding biological structures is stored in a suitable form in the computer. Various methods can then be used to transform these data in order to display the desired information in a variety of ways useful to teaching. Such a system could be used to view structures on command with a variety of orientations. A beginning has already been made on this project at M.I.T.: the computer is used to produce three dimensional drawings of some of the cell groups in the superior-olivary complex in the cat's brain stem. Serial sections, alternately stained with cresyl violet and with protargol, are examined, and the outlines of the important cell groups are traced. These outlines are read into a computer that can then produce stereoscopic or projection drawings on the collections of these outlines.

Certain laboratory tests that require visual examination of cell preparations may be automated by using a digital computer. Work in progress is leading to several methods for performing differential leukocyte counts. One of these techniques, based on examining the scattered light from a cell, may lead to an economical system for automating such a test. Procedures using a digital computer are likely to be more reliable and may be extended to detection of pathological leukocytes, screening Papanicolau smears, doing red blood cell indices, and may lead eventually to procedures for the automatic screening of such complex images as chest roentgenograms. Additional work on the clinical aspects, the engineering techniques, and the formal methods is still needed.

Besides such automated analysis, one can use the computer in a variety of ways to improve the quality of visual images now used by the clinician or researcher. For example, through the use of electronic subtraction for change detection, it may be possible to increase the resolution on cerebral arteriograms to the point where small arterioles can be seen. Also contrast enhancement and noise reduction may be possible in electron microscopy.

A replacement for the indirect fundus camera is now under discussion in work done at M.I.T. and the Massachusetts Eye and Ear Infirmary. This would involve a holographic opthalmoscope that provides a larger field of view, gives better resolution, minimizes patient discomfort, and allows stereoscopic viewing. By photographing the wavefront obtained from a brief examination of the patient, the physician can sit down at his leisure and view the reconstructed holographic image just as if he were examining the fundus of his patient, checking all four quadrants in turn merely by changing his angle of viewing.

The technical prerequisites for developing the kinds of sophisticated hardware noted above need strong emphasis. Computer-generated holograms, the effects of noise in the Fourier transforms of a picture, and the development of software are all areas in which work is proceeding. Such an effort is greatly facilitated when it occurs in a setting that allows free collaboration with teaching hospitals, academic departments, and special centers and laboratories. Besides the senior research staff, postdoctoral workers, and students, a number of programmers, technicians, and supporting personnel are needed. A good computing facility and some kind of laboratory space for scanner development, electron microscopy, and the like are also required. Because of the rich resources in these areas present in the M.I.T. complex, a collaborative effort involving these two institutions would seem ideally suited to fruitful research work in the image-processing area.

Task Group Report on Medical Care Microsystems

G. Octo Barnett
DIRECTOR OF THE LABORATORY OF COMPUTER SCIENCE
MASSACHUSETTS GENERAL HOSPITAL, CHAIRMAN

Peter G. Katona
ASSISTANT PROFESSOR OF ELECTRICAL ENGINEERING
MASSACHUSETTS INSTITUTE OF TECHNOLOGY

John F. Rockart
ASSISTANT PROFESSOR OF MANAGEMENT
SLOAN SCHOOL OF MANAGEMENT
MASSACHUSETTS INSTITUTE OF TECHNOLOGY

Herbert Sherman
LINCOLN LABORATORY
MASSACHUSETTS INSTITUTE OF TECHNOLOGY

Health-care delivery may be divided into a number of different areas. To make the massive constellation of health problems manageable, if not soluble, it is necessary to break them apart. Yet solutions to any particular problem in health care delivery are clearly dependent on the status of the other parts of the whole.

Geographically and historically, a hospital may be considered a health care entity, a microsystem within the total system. However, a viable treatment of the hospital as a microsystem must recognize its interdependence on a great many other micro- and macrosystems. Distinctions, for example, between in-hospital and out-of-hospital services are no longer very useful; they result more from accident than systematic planning. In another section of this report, health care macrosystems are explored in depth.

The hospital itself is a complex institution with a conglomeration of hierarchical functions operating in partial isolation from each other. Such functions include patient transportation, the planning of staff schedules, transportation of materials, and inventory control. We have chosen to focus this report on the information processing activities, partly because of the importance this activity has in the institution's total functioning, and partly because it appears to represent a promising area for improvement through technological innovation.

Information processing is of fundamental importance to the patient care process. Although the volume of information used in medical care has increased substantially, there have been few improvements in the handling of this information. Most of the information is written, often in illegible script, on multipart forms. The same information must be delivered to many different areas in the hospital by multiple slips of paper or a number of telephone calls. Most of the information is retrieved by shuffling through stacks of reports or leafing through the medical record—a rather disorganized collection of doctors' and nurses' observations, test results, and records of therapeutic activities. A recent study of hospital costs has shown that over 25 percent of a hospital's budget is spent on information processing.[1] Furthermore, a significant and costly portion of the time of the physician, nurse, and technical staff, is taken up by bookkeeping activities.

The main theme of this report is the potential for the application of technology to information processing. However, we would emphasize that innovations in health care, technical or otherwise, face the same tests of feasibility that confront changes in other fields. We applaud a closer integration of medicine and technology, but we recognize that acceptance of the political and social realities surrounding the task of implementing new ideas or techniques demands that the clinical-technical alliance be broadened to include the systems analyst, the industrial management engineer, the sociologist, the economist, the political scientist, and perhaps the politician, among others.

In analyzing information processing needs, it is operationally misleading to speak in terms of a total hospital information system. The most productive tactic appears to be the development of modules for specific information processing activities, allowing precise identification of objectives and requirements. Further, the modular approach facilitates the introduction of new technology into an existing health care system that must continue to function. On the other hand, the modules cannot be planned and implemented *in vacuo*. Attention must be given to an over-all framework and the integration of component units.

To present the dimensions of the information processing area, five examples of modules are described. In each case we give a brief general description of the problem area and its potential for technological innovation. We conclude with a discussion of the effort required for appropriate research and development and criteria for assigning priorities to the various modules. The five areas are: (1) laboratory data processing; (2) medical records; (3) medical histories; (4) medical diagnosis; and (5) hospital communication systems.

Laboratory Data Processing

The clinical laboratory is one of the few well-defined information processing tasks in the hospital. It is also probably the area where most effort has been exerted to develop automated systems for information processing. There are several reasons for this. Significant improvements in the handling of laboratory test information

TASK GROUP REPORT ON MEDICAL CARE MICROSYSTEMS

may be made independently of other hospital information processing tasks. The need for faster and more accurate data handling in the laboratory is great: the workload has been doubling every five to seven years, and scarce, trained lab personnel now spend 50 percent of their time recording, transcribing, and reporting test data.

The computer can be useful in the clinical laboratory in a number of ways. An automated data processing system can provide, for example, specimen identification, automatic reading of instrumentation, conversion of raw results to reportable units, quality control and monitoring of the instrumentation itself, compilation and generation of laboratory data reports, and production of laboratory test result summaries for each patient. Computer techniques are useful in detecting in laboratory data, unusual clinical patterns in which the presence of an abnormality may be signified by a combination of several test results rather than by a change in a single test.

To develop criteria for adapting any proposed system to the needs of particular laboratory installations, a number of issues must be considered. Among these are economy, scale, degree of centralization, communication requirements, quantity and variety of tests performed, and the kinds of instrumentation utilized. Just as third generation computer operating systems are modular and expandable to meet particular configuration requirements, a modular and expandable laboratory information system needs to be designed. A substantial commitment of technical personnel and resources is required to develop system specifications to meet the spectrum of existing needs. Most industrial or research efforts to date have been responsive mainly to ad hoc needs or have been aimed at a particular market. Neither industry nor individual research projects are likely to commit themselves to an undertaking of the size needed. The situation is somewhat parallel to the experience in developing the LINC, a small general-purpose digital computer especially designed to meet the need for a laboratory instrument for the medical investigator. The development was an N.I.H.-sponsored activity carried out by a university-affiliated group to fulfill a clear-cut need that industry had largely failed to recognize. Once developed, the

LINC was produced commercially and stimulated a whole series of further computer developments by industry for this market. Similarly, in developing automated information systems for the clinical laboratory, it appears necessary to define objectives more clearly, to develop prototype units, and to induce industry to implement them.

Medical Records

Current use of medical records suffers from a number of basic deficiencies. First, records are often illegible and disorganized and reflect the skills, interests, and mannerisms of individual physicians. The records are not indexed and have no standard form. Without tedious record review, information is often lost to follow-up. Even when found, the data are subject to various interpretations. For retrospective record research and review, these retrieval problems are compounded by orders of magnitude.

Collecting clinical information in a form that permits retrieval and analysis by computer holds a long sought potential for evaluating the nature of disease, the reliability of diagnostic procedures, and the efficacy of treatments, i.e., for auditing the medical care process. The Professional Activities Study (PAS) [2] provides a system for processing discharge summaries from a number of participating hospitals and generating reports indicating various statistics on diagnoses, laboratory values, and so on, for the hospitals' use. The Permanente Medical Group administers a voluntary prepaid multiphasic screening program for the periodic, routine health examination of its members, and by accumulating a data base through follow-up studies over a period of years, it is in a unique position to evaluate the efficacy of a number of routine diagnostic procedures in screening for disease.[3] Other isolated efforts of the sort have also met with moderate success.

The retrieval of clinical information depends on how the data are structured. The possibility of free text retrieval seems to be limited to those portions of the record that are sufficiently narrow in context that a synonym dictionary or thesaurus can serve this purpose. Levy, Cammarn, and Smith and Lamson [4] have, for example, experimented with automating input and retrieval of pathology reports in natural language form. Methods such as that of Allen [5] provide versatile on-line storage and retrieval capabilities for use with more structured data files.

Because of the richness of the language of clinical medicine and the very limited nature of the automated syntactical and semantic analysis techniques available, it is neither feasible nor desirable to emulate on the computer system the human being's natural language processing capabilities and pattern recognition skills. Retrieval of information in this form is expensive, inefficient and often inaccurate because of problems of semantic interpretation.

At the other extreme, all possible inputs to the computer system might be anticipated by an exhaustive check list that permits concise coding and efficient, economical search and retrieval. This would guarantee a well-defined, unambiguous vocabulary and permit the imposition of a significant degree of quality control at the time of input. However, this approach often requires excessive time and effort and imposes what may be unacceptable restrictions on the user's freedom of expression. The medical record represents especially difficult problems in this regard because of the wide variety and complexity of information it contains and the relatively free and unstructured holographic form in which it is traditionally recorded.

A promising approach is the use of the computer and an interactive terminal device to facilitate the information-gathering process by means of a branching question-answer dialogue between the user and the computer. Much of the information currently recorded in the medical record is not really unconstrained free text at all but rather patterned statements that the physician usually uses to describe particular ideas. A branching dialogue with a computer may facilitate this process by permitting the physician to select very quickly the topics he wishes to discuss. These topics may be expanded in further displays, and material not relevant to the current problem may be bypassed. The use of structured displays and directed conversation not only provides standardization of terminology but also has educational values: a display may remind a physician to review otherwise neglected topics.

A structured medical record would have significant advantages for comprehensive medical care systems, since it would be much easier for health personnel to evaluate a patient's total health needs if his data were assembled and presented in a concise, well-ordered, and unambiguous fashion.

Applying these techniques to capture clinical information involves simultaneous and coordinated activity in at least four areas involving both medical and technical resources:

A. The development of generally accepted, medically precise, and useful subject material for structuring the information in specific clinical areas. This will require concerted effort by a large number of medical specialists in selecting appropriate terminology and organizing and evaluating it.

B. The design of low-cost remote display and hard copy input-output devices. Because of the dependence on interactive dialogue in which a large amount of stylized material is available to be presented to the physician, there is great dependence on a remote rapid display device such as an alphanumeric display scope or a "random access" film strip projector. Indeed, the economics involved will no doubt be the major limiting factor in the wise dissemination of this approach.

C. Design of large-scale data-management systems suitable for handling hierarchically structured files of clinical data. Mass storage and slow random-access capability are required in a system that attempts to provide continuity and comprehensiveness by means of a centralized clinical data base. The extent to which networks of this type are feasible, desirable, or economically practical must be considered. The usefulness of large computer utilities, such as MULTICS, for this problem should receive attention.

D. The development of problem-oriented languages for controlling computer-user dialogues, for data-base manipulation, and for report generation. A class of programming subsystems must be developed to support the input, file handling, and retrieval of clinical data, largely because of its rather complex chronological as well as topical organization.

Work in this area can have significant long-term effects on the nature of medical practice, its teaching, and its body of knowledge. The great increase in specialization among physicians and the use of paramedical personnel in the delivery of care has shifted a good deal of responsibility for continuity of care from the family doctor to the medical record.

Medical Histories

In the current practice of medicine, obtaining a patient's history is usually the first stage of the patient encounter. This doctor-patient dialogue may have one or more goals. If a patient comes with a specific complaint, a series of questions will be directed at determining specifically the possible causes of the symptom. If a patient comes with a known disease, the questions may be directed at determining the status of the disease and its progression. In the case of an annual or periodic checkup, the goal is to screen for the presence or absence of a number of important signs and symptoms that may indicate the early stages of disease.

Recording patient histories in this fashion may take a physician as little as one or two minutes or as much as an hour. In each instance he chooses a series of appropriate questions from a very large set, the selections being based on the patient's responses to previous questions. The quality of the history depends on the physician's logic patterns, his memory, and the time he can devote to the process. Increasing demands on the physician's time and an exponential rise in the amount and complexity of data known about disease have both had a deleterious effect on the quality of histories obtained. There have been, therefore, several attempts to develop ancillary methods for the acquisition of patient histories.

The first attempts used printed questionnaires and were limited by the number of questions that could be put on a form. In addition, this technique did not use the physician's branching logic to determine the specific questions set for each patient.

Both automation and time-sharing have made it possible to simulate more closely some of the physician's techniques. With either a CRT or teletypewriter as a remote terminal, these experimental programs present a series of questions to the patient, with a number of answer choices. Each question is based on the answer to previous questions, using a branching technique similar to the physician's. At the conclusion of the dialogue at the terminal, a summary of the information acquired is printed out for the physician's use in evaluating the case.

Research in the use of automated medical histories has for several reasons expanded very slowly. Medical expertise needed for content development is difficult to obtain, and to date, experiments with automated histories have covered only small areas of content. Work has been redundant with different groups covering essentially the same content area. Further, implementation of automated history taking is currently very expensive; the cost of communication and of terminals has severely handicapped research and development. Until low-cost terminals and relatively inexpensive, remote access, computer systems are available, it is doubtful that experimentation with this technique will go very far.

Results of the few experiments with automated medical histories have been generally positive. Patients and physicians both seem to like the technique, and clearly it has the potential for saving physician's time. However, a thorough evaluation of the automated history-taking procedure is still lacking. In fact, the significance of the medical history within the medical record and of the whole medical record in the practice of medicine has not been satisfactorily examined and established. A thorough appraisal of automated techniques in the delivery of patient care thus depends on the development of appropriate and useful theories and methods of measuring the quality of medical care in general.

Medical Diagnosis

A number of experiments with computer aids to clinical decision-making have been carried out, usually applying Bayes' Theorem to diagnosis in a relatively circumscribed clinical area. Other efforts have dealt with the use of factor analysis, multivariate analysis, likelihood functions, or various heuristics. The major difficulty in extending these efforts to larger subsets of problems has been the lack of good data on which to base the estimates of probabilities, weights, or heuristics. It is our opinion that the pursuit of computer-aided diagnosis will remain largely theoretical for some time and that the problem area could not be greatly advanced by a large scale-up of effort. The major advances will probably come from smaller-scale commitments by individual investigation or of small groups of investigators. Automated medical record systems, by providing good clinical data, will ultimately be of great use in this area; at present, however, it seems to warrant a rather modest commitment by individual investigators.

Specific diagnostic processes, on the other hand, seem ripe for immediate pursuit. In electrocardiographic analysis, there are a number of technical as well as theoretical questions to be solved, and good data on which to base diagnostic criteria are available. There are at least two conflicting approaches to the problems of ECG recording and morphological identification; arrhythmia analysis has only recently begun to receive attention; and there are as yet no commercial systems available to the medical profession that can carry out ECG interpretation in an acceptable fashion. It would appear, therefore, that this particular area of diagnosis might be a suitable subject for investigation.

Hospital Communication Systems

The application of computers to patient care that is of greatest interest to commercial computer firms has been labeled "Hospital Information Systems" (HIS). To the physician, this means a system that will provide rapid, accurate, and legible communication of reports, better scheduling procedures, and timely and precise implementation of activities ordered for patient care. To the nurse HIS implies an operation to lighten the clerical load in preparing requisitions and transcribing and charting. To the administrator HIS is a means for using resources more effectively, for gathering the data necessary for appropriate management decision, and for ensuring that information necessary to the patient billing process is readily available and accurate. By all odds the development of automated hospital information systems is one of the most complex and difficult areas in the data processing field, and the comments below merely suggest a few points of concern. Numerous studies indicate that almost all the information processing activity related to patient care on a hospital ward is the direct or indirect result of doctors' orders. Doctors' orders are instructions written by physicians to initiate actions by doctors, nurses, or paramedical personnel for a specific patient. They are recorded and transcribed many times and affect every hospital department or service. A hospital information system designed to reflect this relationship should be developed and tested.

The major emphasis in the development of hospital communication systems has been in the use of a real-time, on-line computer system with multiple input/output terminals located in patient care units and in all service areas. There are a few research projects involved in this area, including several sponsored directly by the computer industry. The principle technical problems concern: (a) the lack of appropriate, inexpensive terminals; (b) the requirement for a very reliable time-sharing, multiterminal computer system with flexible programming support; and (c) the need to have a rather large support group of system analysts, computer programmers, and engineers. An equally critical problem is the need for a major commitment and allocation of resources from the medical facility where the development is being undertaken. Developmental efforts must be concerned not only with technology but also with considerations of how to test and evaluate communication systems in existing institutions.

Thus far, most successful efforts have been with relatively isolated and small-scale projects. This is owing partly to the fact that every existing research project in this area has had the resources to attack only a limited subset of problems and partly because the supporting technology has been so inadequate. At the present rate, at least a decade will be required to develop the variety of systems needed. With HIS, as with other particularly complex information processing problems, it may well be that a modular approach is the only feasible and effective method of attack.

Conclusion

Significant improvements in the health care delivery system are now at hand through the application of technology. A few have been suggested in this report. As medical care comes increasingly under national scrutiny, the need for a more efficient, less expensive and more reliable health system and for standards to measure them is increasingly apparent. Technology's role in achieving better health systems is clear and must be exploited with a new and greater commitment of medical, technical, and financial resources.

Within the university communities of Harvard and the Massachusetts Institute of Technology, there is a high degree of interest in developing a cooperative effort aimed at this need. What is lacking is a suitable organizational framework within which the clinician and technologist may work. We propose, therefore, the establishment of a new institute, sponsored jointly by Harvard Medical School and its affiliated hospitals and M.I.T., and dedicated to these objectives:

1. To delineate problems in health care delivery that are soluble through the application of technology.
2. To develop methods and techniques for solving these problems.
3. To test the new technology as prototype activities within existing health care institutions.
4. To assist other medical facilities and industry in replicating the successful prototypes.

A number of factors demand the creation of a new agency, one with a firm academic base. The most critical of these is that to attract and hold top flight medical personnel, affiliation with a medical institution is essential. On the other hand, neither the medical school nor a hospital is an appropriate base for the strong technical staff necessary for an applications-oriented technological mission. To maintain channels for replication of the institute's developments and inventions, it will be necessary to have a close relationship with private industry and a variety of other health-related institutions that may not be indigenous to the academic environment.

The institute is envisioned, then, as a financially and administratively independent organization, staffed by a core of full-time investigators and by faculty from the sponsoring institutions. Graduate students and medical students should be able to use the institute's facilities either for research or to participate in ongoing institute projects.

Several important criteria will identify the appropriate constellation of problems for the institute to tackle: the time required to achieve marketable results; the immediacy of the need for the change; and the scale of effort involved. The institute should take seriously the question of an appropriate division of responsibility among academic research, industrial research and development, and its own efforts. Projects should be divided between those with promise of a relatively quick payoff (e.g., clinical laboratory systems) and those that will require a more massive and long-term investment (e.g., medical record systems).

In every case, a balance must be struck between developing applications independent of a specific geographic need and developing applications that will command the endorsement of specific institutions. In fact, hospital and medical leadership should be involved in the institute at its highest policy-making and control levels—the board of directors.

Some present M.I.T.-Harvard Medical School cooperative efforts are restrained by a lack of optimal test facilities for new engineering developments Considerations of cost and limited resources, among others, overrule the establishment of new facilities for testing; besides, the true challenge is to develop techniques that can be implemented in existing medical care systems. One reason the institute's developmental efforts will need strong independent financial support is to keep the cost from becoming an impediment to participation of a hospital or other facility.

The high cost of medical-technical research and development has been mentioned several times in this discussion. Financing of the institute's work must be commensurate with the magnitude of the problems under study and stable enough to support long-range problem solving and researchers of outstanding caliber. Control of the funding should rest within the institute, allowing it to recruit and support talented individuals from medicine and technology wherever they are located. Based on an estimate of the manpower and hardware needed to carry on the five projects reviewed in this report, the institute's budget for a year will approximate two-and-one-half to three million dollars (twenty full-time equivalent senior staff and sixty supporting technical and clerical staff). The institute should, we feel, be housed within an easy distance of the sponsoring universities; on the other hand, some projects could (and should) be housed outside of institute grounds.

The institute should be committed to having its prototype units replicated and, therefore, to development by private industry of these units as commercial products. Private industry has hesitated to enter this field partly because it lacks a definable market, so the institute should bring together potential users of its new technology for intensive indoctrination and training. In sum, the institute would define the nature of the problem, develop and test the prototype model, work with industry to have this model developed, educate the user community in order to facilitate initial marketing of the industrial product, and maintain a program of continuing education by serving as a distribution point for information, user group activity, and quality control of the industrial product. At the same time, close contact with medical practice will be necessary to keep the institute aware of changing needs and practices in health-care delivery and stimulate it to update prototype models on a continuing basis.

Many of the important roadblocks to improving the health-care delivery system are not technological in the classical sense but are rather problems of management and allocation of resources, relating to the health care power structure and the need for area-wide planning. Representation in the institute of people from the social sciences, economics, law, operations research, industrial management, business administration, and education is, therefore, extremely desirable.

Footnotes

[1] R. A. Jydstrup and M. J. Gross, "Cost of Information Handling in Hospitals," *Health Service Research* 1 (Winter 1966) : 235–271.

[2] V. N. Slee, "Information Systems and Measurement Tools," *Journal of the American Medical Association* 196 (June 20, 1966) : 1063–1065.

[3] M. F. Collen, "Periodic Health Examinations Using an Automated Multitest Laboratory," *Journal of the American Medical Association* 195 (March 7, 1966) : 830–833.

[4] R. P. Levy, M. R. Cammarn, and M. J. Smith, "Computer Handling of Ambulatory Clinic Records," *Journal of the American Medical Association* 190 (December 21, 1964) : 1033–1037.

[5] S. I. Allen, G. O. Barnett, and P. A. Castleman, "Use of a Time-shared General-purpose File-handling System in Hospital Research," *Proceedings of IEEE* 54 (December, 1966) : 1641–1648.

Task Group Report on Neurophysiology

Nelson Y. Kiang
DIRECTOR OF RESEARCH AT EATON-PEABODY LABORATORY
MASSACHUSETTS EYE AND EAR INFIRMARY, CHAIRMAN

Adelbert Ames III
ASSOCIATE BIOCHEMIST, DEPARTMENT OF NEUROSURGERY
MASSACHUSETTS GENERAL HOSPITAL

Charles F. Barlow
BRONSON CROTHERS PROFESSOR OF NEUROLOGY & HEAD OF DEPARTMENT
OF NEUROLOGY
CHILDREN'S HOSPITAL MEDICAL CENTER

John S. Barlow
NEUROPHYSIOLOGIST, DEPARTMENT OF NEUROLOGY
MASSACHUSETTS GENERAL HOSPITAL

David H. Hubel
PROFESSOR OF NEUROPHYSIOLOGY, DEPARTMENT OF NEUROBIOLOGY
HARVARD MEDICAL SCHOOL

Stephen W. Kuffler
ROBERT WINTHROP PROFESSOR OF NEUROBIOLOGY AND
HEAD OF DEPARTMENT OF NEUROBIOLOGY
HARVARD MEDICAL SCHOOL

William T. Peake
ASSOCIATE PROFESSOR OF ELECTRICAL ENGINEERING
RESEARCH LABORATORY OF ELECTRONICS
MASSACHUSETTS INSTITUTE OF TECHNOLOGY

Kenneth N. Stevens
PROFESSOR OF ELECTRICAL ENGINEERING
RESEARCH LABORATORY OF ELECTRONICS
MASSACHUSETTS INSTITUTE OF TECHNOLOGY

Torsten N. Wiesel
PROFESSOR OF PHYSIOLOGY, DEPARTMENT OF NEUROBIOLOGY
HARVARD MEDICAL SCHOOL

Thomas F. Weiss
ASSOCIATE PROFESSOR OF ELECTRICAL ENGINEERING
RESEARCH LABORATORY OF ELECTRONICS
MASSACHUSETTS INSTITUTE OF TECHNOLOGY

Neurophysiological research in the Harvard-M.I.T. complex today is found in many places. These research units have widely different interests and capabilities. The present report is an attempt to determine whether there might be useful consequences of closer cooperation between these units and what directions such cooperation might take. Although we shall limit our discussions to Harvard Medical School, its associated hospitals, and M.I.T., there are other institutions in the Boston area that could also have been included.

Traditionally, neurophysiological research has been concentrated in medical schools and biology departments. More recently, though, this field has attracted the interest of workers trained predominantly in disciplines such as the physical sciences, communication sciences, or psychology. Typically, workers in one field have not taken formal training in the others, so it is to be expected that gaps in communication should develop. Despite the many so-called interdisciplinary conferences, these gaps still exist, with the result that neurophysiology in the Boston area is still characterized by small clusters of isolated efforts. An explosive increase in technical capability and the resulting diversity of expertise have contributed to fragmentation.

It can be argued that a pluralistic approach is more desirable than a single coordinated attack; and indeed, there are some first-rate scientists who prefer to work in small, isolated groups. Nonetheless, many opportunities for useful interactions between groups of similar inclinations at M.I.T. and Harvard have doubtless gone unrecognized.

This committee agrees that interaction between those trained in the biological and medical sciences and those in the physical and engineering sciences can be mutually profitable. However, the heavy pressures of present duties leave little time to develop such associations, and it seems unrealistic to expect that large numbers of established investigators will have either the time or flexibility to develop new and different attitudes. Encourage such explorations in students is an excellent idea, but at present there are few opportunities for students to receive formal training in neurophysiology except by working in a specific laboratory. There are virtually no graduate courses in neurophysiology offered at either institution and nothing that even remotely resembles a program of studies. Teaching in this field is still essentially by the apprentice system, a factor that contributes to the insular outlook of many workers in neurophysiology.

It should be possible from the wealth of talent available in the Boston area to establish courses or seminars in such fields as neuroanatomy, neurophysiology, neurochemistry, biophysics, communication sciences, psychophysics, and physiological psychology that which would be open to qualified students from any institution. This way students with very different backgrounds would have a common core of formal training to carry into their future research projects. These students could then concentrate their efforts in their chosen areas without being totally ignorant of more general areas of related knowledge.

There is also a consensus in this committee that lasting and significant cooperation cannot be established in the atmosphere of a crash program. Rather there must be an evolutionary process with time for the participants to develop solid working relationships. Thus there is little enthusiasm for a massive influx of funds to support central research facilities or institute-like configurations —although this may develop with time and experience. As a start, one could hope for the establishment of a clearing house for information on existing resources and research programs. This information should be kept current and made available to students. A strong attempt should be made to develop an introductory neural sciences course that would provide a broad survey of the fields and introduce students to active workers in specialized areas. More specialized courses could then be offered by individuals or groups as they wished, without being concerned about overlapping coverage. These courses should not be disjointed series of lectures but should strive to present consistent viewpoints. A course on membrane physiology given by an electrical engineer might well be very different from one offered by a molecular biologist, but the student should have the opportunity to become familiar with both approaches. Financial support should be available to applicants who can demonstrate competence in their area and a specific plan for teaching. Such support might be used for teaching assistants, development of teaching materials, and laboratory supplies and equipment.

As various courses are developed in the basic neural sciences, there should be a parallel development of courses in clinical neurophysiology. At present the accumulated knowledge in areas such as neurology, neurosurgery, otolaryngology, and opthalmology is available almost exclusively to physicians and surgeons. There should be opportunities for graduate students to gain some familiarity with clinical problems. Hopefully this experience would open some channels of communication between clinicians and research workers in the basic sciences.

Eventually there may be need to provide special space to train students, but it is difficult to assess the extent of this need at the present time.

Initially the total cost of maintaining a clearing house and developing a set of introductory and intermediate courses would be $50,000 per year. If successful, the cost would become significantly greater as more students are attracted and more faculty are required.

In summary, the greatest need in neurophysiology today is well-trained neurophysiologists. We suggest that efforts be exerted to encourage formal teaching and that some attempt be made to develop a coordinated interinstitutional program. Hopefully this effort will in itself result in the development of mutual respect and understanding among the students if not the faculty. Through this step a firm basis for intellectual interaction among research groups at Harvard and M.I.T. will be established, and it may be that proposals for specific collaborative research will result. Those research projects in which collaboration already exists can only be strengthened by the addition of a common goal in teaching.

Task Group Report on Organ and Cell Culture and Storage

Sanford A. Miller
ASSOCIATE PROFESSOR OF NUTRITION
MASSACHUSETTS INSTITUTE OF TECHNOLOGY, CHAIRMAN

Ernest G. Cravalho
ASSISTANT PROFESSOR OF MECHANICAL ENGINEERING
MASSACHUSETTS INSTITUTE OF TECHNOLOGY

Harvey M. Shein
PSYCHIATRIST
McLEAN HOSPITAL

Anthony J. Sinskey
ASSISTANT PROFESSOR OF NUTRITION
MASSACHUSETTS INSTITUTE OF TECHNOLOGY

Daniel I. C. Wang
ASSISTANT PROFESSOR OR NUTRITION
MASSACHUSETTS INSTITUTE OF TECHNOLOGY

Introduction

The thrust of modern medicine is no more evident than in the attempt to establish *in vitro* models and systems equivalent to those existing in the living organism. The use of tissue culture techniques has allowed the researcher to isolate and study a number of vital aspects of the living system. Unfortunately, the fruits of this fundamental approach to the complexities of the living system have not become widely available in the practice of medicine. For the most part, this has been because of the enormous difficulties and great skills required to successfully culture most of the cell lines of interest. The result has been the avoidance of the use of these techniques by many investigators.

In a real sense, the position of the technique is similar to that of the use of whole animals at the start of the century or the use of enzymes during the thirties in that each investigator has had to develop his own techniques for maintaining his colony or preparing his enzyme before being able to perform his studies. Thus an inordinate amount of time was spent on matters not directly concerned with the major problem. Today the availability of commercial breeders and the development of suppliers of biological materials have played important roles in the enormous increase in studies using these materials. Nothing of the sort, however, has yet occurred in the practice of tissue and organ culture.

The lack of widespread availability of cells and organs has also resulted in the number of cell lines being limited since most workers are not concerned with research in developing new lines. The tremendous research required to isolate and determine the requirements for survival of new cell lines has been instrumental in preventing increases in the number of lines available for research. Moreover, the lack of large-scale devices has discouraged use of tissue culture for the direct production of materials useful in medical practice, e.g., hormones and antibodies.

The problem of storage of cells and organs has also not received the attention it requires. The problem of organ storage is particularly acute: recent successes in the area of organ transplantation have depended upon the availability of compatible donors. Since the timing of the transplant is of vital significance to the success of the procedure, both legal and moral issues have been raised regarding the haste with which the organs are removed from the donor. It is obvious that much of this concern could be removed if techniques and facilities were available for the storage of organs and cell structures. It would be possible to remove the vital organ with no problem of doubt as to the death of the donor. At the present time, neither the techniques nor the facilities are available.

The need for the development of large-scale tissue culture techniques has become obvious; the need for development and availability of new cell lines suitable for research are equally apparent; and the requirement of long-term storage of cells and organs in such ventures is obvious. For these reasons, the establishment of a center to provide research in those areas not currently being pursued is proposed. This center would have as its principal mission the study of methods of tissue culture and storage rather than that of cell systems. Its goals would be as follows: (a) to develop the technology suitable for the growth of cells in large quantities; (b) to develop new cell lines of interest to and required by scientists working in the field; (c) to provide cells on a contract basis for other workers; (d) to develop a suitable technology for the use of cells in the production of products of medical interest; (e) to develop the techniques necessary for the storage of cells and organs; (f) to study the integration of cells into organs in terms of their function.

Problem Areas

MASS CELL CULTURE

The most obvious area of interaction, certainly the area most important for development, is that of mass cell culture. The production of large amounts of cells of a variety of types would allow the investigator more time to pursue the central theme of his studies. Moreover, the development of such techniques would provide a framework upon which the development of cell types capable of producing products of immediate medical interest could be built. These could include the production of vaccines, enzymes, antibodies, and hormones. Using the last product as an example, if it became possible to propagate in pure culture and in large quantities the cell type in the anterior pituitary that synthesizes human somatotrophic hormone, a rich but inexpensive source of the material would be available for clinical use. In addition, the growth of specific lymphocytes for cancer chemotherapy could provide another area of fruitful research. Cells produced in this center would also be used for, say, understanding of the mechanism by which neurons operate, metabolism of tumor cells, development of lymphoid cells and their role in antibody production, studies of the mechanism of tissue rejection in transplantation procedures, and the synthesis of hormones.

The problems associated with mass culture are, in part, those of engineering a biological system. They include the question of appropriate materials, methods of aeration, centrifugation, flow, and so on. To these must be added the specific complexities of the animal cell. For example, the lack of a cell wall makes collection of cells difficult. The problem of deformation under conditions of fast flow also must be considered. Some background for this work can be obtained from the project at Roswell Park in Buffalo, New York, where an attempt to develop large-scale production of a single type of cell is now in progress. Even in this case, however, the lack of an effective, intimate, and continuing relationship between engineers and life scientists has made the project difficult to accomplish.

PURE CULTURE TECHNIQUES

Present techniques for cultivation of differentiated cell types from a given tissue or organ employ either explants of tissue from that organ or dispersed cell cultures derived by enzyme treatment of tissue from the organ. Explants or dispersed cell cultures prepared by these standard techniques include mixtures of the many different histological cell types. In order to obtain a pure cell culture consisting exclusively of a single, differentiated cell type, further procedures are required to separate the desired cell type from the other histological cell types. At present this separation can in some instances be accomplished by cloning, i.e., by isolating a single cell of the desired type under conditions that permit: (1) subsequent serial multiplication *in vitro* of the desired cell type and (2) retention of differentiated characteristics of the cell type among the progeny that arise via its further multiplication *in vitro*.

Among normal cell types, only those have been cultivated in pure culture that can be readily cloned, then readily identified by *in vitro* chemical or histochemical tests. For example, cartilage cells, striated muscle cells, and retinal pigment cells—all cell types easily identifiable by unique morphological characteristics—have been grown in pure culture by these techniques. However, most histological cell types, including those of greatest potential medical interest, exhibit inadequate growth potential or sufficiently distinctive morphological and functional characteristics for certain identification *in vitro* by present techniques and thus have not been cloned. In addition, many of these cell types exhibit morphological and functional "de-differentiation" *in vitro* when cultured in isolation from other cell types of the organ of origin, so the identity of these cell types could not be determined at present even assuming that cloning were achieved and that reliable *in vitro* identifying criteria were available for that cell type.

A number of classical studies on nutritional and growth requirements of isolated normal cells *in vitro* have established that different, differentiated cell types exhibit specific, very fastidious requirements for substances in the nutrient medium and in the microenvironment in addition to the usual balanced salts, amino acids, vitamins, and serum. In the absence of these specific substances, the cell type may survive in an explanted organ but will not survive in a differentiated form capable of further multiplication *in vitro* after isolation from the organ. For example, neurons from sympathetic ganglia survive in explants for days or even weeks *in vitro* without adding a highly specific protein nerve growth factor (NGF); but in dispersed cell culture these neurons will not survive for more than a day without addition of NGF.

Some further conception of the primitive state of presently available techniques for pure cell cultivation may be conveyed by listing some of the medically important, histologically differentiated cell types that have not yet been propagated in pure culture: brain cell types (neurons; oligodendrocytes, astrocytes); endocrine cell types (of every known type); lymphocytes (only very limited multiplication of partially purified cell population has been achieved); thymocytes and bone marrow cell types; and parenchymal cell types from liver, kidney, heart, lung, and skin.

Availability of pure cell cultures of different brain cell types would for the first time make possible biochemical and biophysical studies to determine the distinctive structural components and distinctive enzyme complements of neurons, astrocytes and oligodendrocytes. Studies of the effects of different neurohumors, hormones, and psychotropic drugs on these cultures would provide basic data relevant to brain cell plasticity, growth migration, and regeneration. Availability of pure cell cultures of different endocrine cell types would make possible definitive analyses of factors controlling the synthesis, storage, and release of the various hormones. Availability of pure cell cultures of differentiated plasma cells, lymphocytes, thymocytes, and bone marrow cell types would make possible more detailed experimental analyses of the interactions of these various cell types in self-other recognition, in production and control of cell-bound and humoral antibody, and in protection (immunity) against viruses, bacteria, fungi, and tumor cells. Availability of pure cultures of other parenchymal cell types, e.g., liver or kidney cells, would make possible more detailed analyses, at the molecular level, of factors controlling induction and repression of specific enzymes of medical interest.

It is apparent from the previous discussion of the present status of pure cell cultivation techniques that the techniques for almost all cell types are still in early stages of development. Further developmental research will be required to improve techniques in all the principal problem areas, including procedures for: (a) dispersing cells from tissues, (b) separating different cell types, (c) stimulating continued cell division of the separated cell types *in vitro*, (d) maintaining differentiation of the separated cell types *in vitro*, (e) identifying specific cell types *in vitro* by development of more adequate morphological and functional (biochemical) criteria.

The obvious advantages to the long-term storage of cells and organ systems have already been discussed. It should be sufficient to state that the ultimate functioning and success of the mass production of cells will depend upon the development of appropriate storage techniques. It is also obvious that full realization of the potential of the transplant procedures will also depend upon the solution of the storage problem.

The attainment of a successful storage system will have to occur in three general steps. These are: (a) the solution of the problems associated with the storage of cells for a significant period of time without changing functional capacity; (b) the extension of these results to the exceedingly complex structure of the organ; and (c) the engineering of suitable facilities for the storage of cells and organs.

Specifically, the problem areas associated with cell storage include:

1. Catalog of cell types that make up vital organs.
2. Engineering models of the physical make-up of various cell types.
3. Catalog of the biological and biochemical process in the various types of cells.
4. Interactions between a cell and its environment.
5. Significant environmental parameters and the manner in which they affect cell viability.
6. Tests for cell viability.
7. Thermodynamic properties of cells and cell structures.
8. Determination of lethal factors.
9. Models for the mechanisms by which fatality occurs.
10. Parameters that influence, affect, or control lethal factors.
11. Cell separation techniques.

One very promising method for the preservation and storage of cell cultures and organs involves the use of low temperatures. Associated with this particular storage technique are additional, more detailed questions which must be answered. Among these are:

1. Energy and mass transport processes associated with cooling and freezing biological structures.

2. Energy and mass transport processes associated with warming and thawing biological structures.
3. Effects of cooling and freezing rates on cell viability.
4. Effects of warming and thawing rates on cell viability.
5. Artificial augmentation of freezing and thawing rates by both chemical and mechanical means.
6. Influence of ice structure on cell viability.
7. Effects of temperature on cell viability.

Questions very much like these must also be answered with regard to organ storage, but probably the most important problem in organ storage is that of the role played by the structure of the organ itself. An organ is a heterogeneous structure composed of a number of different cell types. Thus the problem of mass and energy transport through such a structure becomes much more complicated than transport for a single cell type.

Engineering problems that must be resolved include instrumental and hardware design at both the experimental and the application stages. These problems embrace such questions as material compatibility and the need for miniature instrumentation.

Organization and Structure of a Center

The need for a centrally located facility to provide the services discussed earlier is quite apparent. It is important to state again that the chief missions of such a center would not be in studies of the cell as a physiologic entity but rather in the technology of cell growth. Basic studies are inescapable for such investigations, of course, but it is important to emphasize the technological basis of the approach. The center concept is very useful for such an undertaking: the high costs in developing large-scale fermentors and ancillary equipment are too great for any one laboratory. The need for an extensive multidisciplinary group also acts in the favor of a center. In addition, the required intimacy of purpose and thought for such projects also includes housing in a common area, a requirement served only by a center. It is important to restate that this center would in no way compete with existing cell research laboratories. It is the feeling of the committee that existing cell research continue on an individual basis with the center supplying specific cells or technology, but not substituting for the basic research underway. A center of this type would ideally deploy the services of the microbiologist, virologist, cell physiologist, biochemical engineer, biochemist, mechanical and electrical engineer, organ physiologist, physician, and so on. Of the many appropriate geographical areas where such a facility could be established, the greater Boston educational complex, particularly that of M.I.T. and Harvard, would seem the most suitable environment. Not only does this area provide the wealth of talent and variety of disciplines required for the endeavor but the two schools have a long history of mutual attempts to solve a variety of bioengineering and biomedical problems. M.I.T. also provides an academic basis for this research in its training program for biochemical engineers. It is interesting to note that in the development of the Roswell Park installation, the biochemical engineering group at M.I.T. was asked to and, in fact, did act as the principle engineering consultants in the project. Finally, the recent formalization of the many years of informal research cooperation between M.I.T. and Harvard in the Joint Harvard-M.I.T. Committee on Engineering and Living Systems can provide the organizational framework for the formation of the center.

The costs of establishing this center have been variously estimated by members of the committee. For example, the cost of the mass cell culture operation has been estimated by Dr. Wang to be one million dollars for the design and development of a multikiloliter capacity plant with annual operating costs in the order of two-hundred-and-fifty-thousand dollars per year. The pure culture research costs have been estimated to be about three-hundred-thousand while the estimated costs of establishing the organ storage center are about five-hundred thousand dollars. Even considering a significant overlap in requirements, it would appear that excluding the costs of the building and utilities, the cost of establishing a center to perform research in the technology of cell and organ culture and storage is between one million and two million with operating costs in the area of $500,000 per year. It is apparent that part of the costs would have to be shared by the individuals profiting by its operation and using its products; a substantial basic contribution would have to be made.

The value and desirability of the center visualized in this report was apparent. Not only would the medical practitioner profit from the availability of products for therapy at reasonable costs but the researcher would have at hand the raw materials that would allow him to concentrate on his problem, not the technique. The result could be a revolution in research and in the treatment of the ill.

Task Group Report on Physiological Monitoring

Alfred P. Morgan, Jr.
ASSOCIATE IN SURGERY AND INSTRUCTOR IN SURGERY
PETER BENT BRIGHAM HOSPITAL, CHAIRMAN

James Anliker
ACTING CHIEF
BIOELECTRONICS, MEASUREMENTS BRANCH
NASA

Henrik H. Bendixen
ASSISTANT CLINICAL PROFESSOR OF ANESTHESIA
MASSACHUSETTS GENERAL HOSPITAL

Philip N. Bowditch
ASSOCIATE DIRECTOR
INSTRUMENTATION LABORATORY
MASSACHUSETTS INSTITUTE OF TECHNOLOGY

Edward Burger
RESEARCH ASSOCIATE IN PHYSIOLOGY
HARVARD SCHOOL OF PUBLIC HEALTH

Philip A. Drinker
LECTURER IN MEDICAL ENGINEERING
MASSACHUSETTS INSTITUTE OF TECHNOLOGY

Herbert Haessler
DIRECTOR OF RESEARCH
SCIENCE AND ENGINEERING INSTITUTE
WALTHAM, MASSACHUSETTS

James A. Herd
ASSOCIATE IN PHYSIOLOGY
HARVARD MEDICAL SCHOOL

Peter G. Katona
ASSISTANT PROFESSOR OF ELECTRICAL ENGINEERING
MASSACHUSETTS INSTITUTE OF TECHNOLOGY

Bernard Lown
ASSISTANT PROFESSOR OF MEDICINE, DEPARTMENT OF NUTRITION
HARVARD SCHOOL OF PUBLIC HEALTH

Ascher H. Shapiro
CHAIRMAN, DEPARTMENT OF MECHANICAL ENGINEERING
MASSACHUSETTS INSTITUTE OF TECHNOLOGY

Introduction

Members of this task group have met five times. All but one of the meetings were organized as visits to various departments of the institutions represented by committee members where examples of current or completed work relevant to the committee's field—physiological monitoring—have been presented. These presentations (for details see extracts from the minutes at the end of this report) had their own intrinsic interest but also served as starting points for the discussions from which this report is derived.

Most of the members have served on some similar panel, committee, or discussion group in the past, and as a result, our conversations were usually begun with several implicit assumptions. There was also a certain "here we are again" feeling. But as no member would describe himself as a bioengineer, there was hence no precommitment to this field as a potential discipline with its own curriculum, faculty, and degree. Nor could any member be described as a systems analyst or control engineer, although several members have worked closely with them. Much of the committee's final meeting was taken up with a discussion of what this discipline might have to offer the field of physiological monitoring.

Most members have had satisfactory experiences with individual personal collaborations and view kindly the traditional system of ad hoc working relationships, though not all have participated directly in large interinstitutional ventures as have some of the members of the steering committee and the Joint Committee on Engineering and Living Systems (JCELS).

In one sense the members were quite alike: they were drawn from two professions and many specialties, but all were clearly academics. There were neither community practitioners on the medical side nor industrial employees among the engineers.

Nevertheless, these deliberations, or conversations, resulted in at least majority agreement on desirable broad principles of Harvard-M.I.T. association, as well as some particulars concerning the physiologic monitoring field. The principles suggested here are not based on a complete survey of present biology-engineering interactions. Some of the principles and particulars are not supported by objective data beyond the collective experience of the members; their authority is that of personal communication. No apologies are offered for this; a record of weighted opinion and insight is assumed to be a useful committee product.

The early efforts of the committee were directed at defining its purpose. A review of the whole task committee structure and meetings with the other task committee representatives helped in this. However, we also became aware of some of the gaps in the structure. Of these, one area should be mentioned here because of its close relationship to physiologic monitoring: the field of therapeutic devices. The possibility was raised that an additional task committee be created, but this group believes that the field could not be given sufficiently sharp definition to warrant it. The reasons for this are as follows: (a) All of the task committees taking up problems of measurement and diagnosis are concerned with questions that have a fairly firm foundation, both scientifically and medically, directed at gathering and making available information concerning a patient's status. (b) What is then done with this information becomes subject to debate, as therapeutic methods and physical modalities are more subject to individual opinion than other areas of medicine and surgery. There are, of course, many well-established devices and techniques based on engineering technology, such as high voltage or ionizing radiation, but even there the fringes are fuzzy. An example is extracorporeal irradiation, which has been talked about and used to some extent in leukemia therapy and as a method of immunosuppression. Perhaps better examples are the various trackless probes that have been developed for neurosurgery, but are still not widely used by neurosurgeons.

Inevitably, the committee spent some time discussing forms of organization of jointly available resources in biology, medicine, and engineering. This was not completely irrelevant to our primary responsibility, which was to give some definition to the field of physiologic monitoring and to areas of high potential for development. A proposal requires some description of available facilities in which the work can be carried out, and for this reason some assumptions about futue Harvard-M.I.T. association are included.

This report assumes that a new organization will be created, sponsored, and administered jointly by Harvard and M.I.T. Although there are three alternatives (do nothing; act independently; associate), there was general agreement on the third course. It was taken for granted that some translocation of methods and purposes between medicine and engineering is desirable, a question that this committee was surely not formed to examine. It should be noted, however, that the shortcomings of each profession could tend to reinforce the other. One source of public dissatisfaction with technology is fear that efficiency is pursued without regard to social cost; publicly perceived inadequacies of medical services are related to increasing impersonality, specialization, centralization, and inappropriate inclination toward the medical tour de force.

The broad purposes of the new organization (hereafter called the center) are to facilitate application of the engineering sciences to medicine and biology, the providing both faculties with certain services most likely to be attained through joint venture, and above all, education—the primary function of both Harvard and M.I.T. More practically, the goal of planning should be a structure providing flexibility and ability to respond to internal growth stimuli rather than a carefully worded charter. Another objective should be kept in view: the center should study its own operations with considerable formality. Although it is too late for a Harvard-M.I.T. center for engineering and biology to be prototypal, experience gained in operation of a center will in itself be of unusual interest.

The level at which a center might most usefully interact with patient care systems, as presently constituted, is an important consideration in planning the center's possible activity in the monitoring field. It could operate entirely at the laboratory level, for example, or in an entirely abstract "war games" fashion. However, the social and political climate of the times, including the competition for available money, plainly favors an enterprise working close to the delivery of medical services. A second idea in current favor is the concept of regional rather than independent facilities. We believe these are both worthy principles quite apart from whatever appeal they may have to grantors of public funds. But the medical care pyramid is so broad at its base as to be an almost infinite sink for an institution's time, people, and money; it is therefore suggested that the center operate at one level above mass delivery of medical care, at least so far as physiologic monitoring is concerned, in collaboration with clinical study and special care units of the teaching hospitals where a small number of patients are studied and treated as intensively as possible or appropriate. The validation of new or improved techniques, in particular, requires clinical trials in patients about whom maximum collateral information is available. Further, it may bring progress faster to operate at this level: an island of experimental and special activity in the sea of general care creates the contrast that expedites progress.

Locating areas of greatest need in medicine and biology depends on a matter that has not yet been decided: that is, whether or not it is effective or proper in medicine to weigh cost against effectiveness and whether the quality of medical care is measurable in public health terms. For example, if the goal is the longest, most comfortable survival for the largest number of people, it is possible that some presently accepted principles are inconsistent with optimum application of available resources. Obvious examples arise in the intensive care and transplant fields. Application of cost-benefit ratios is impeded somewhat by difficulties in determining the true cost of care, but this is a surmountable accounting problem. A greater difficulty is assigning values to benefits.

Our assumed Harvard-M.I.T. association begins with the policy stratum of a center for biological engineering (in which the JCELS or its successor holds the responsibility for shaping the center's general form and direction) and continues at all levels. The JCELS, acting as trustees, would be expanded to include representatives of the larger community.

The center as a distinct entity has several advantages over a joint academic department or a jointly administered special laboratory. It can seek institutional support in general research support grants and research training program grants. It could have fiscal autonomy and operate its own office of grants and contracts, greatly facilitating transfers of funds and staff salaries between parent institutions. It could define and control its own patent policies—a problem that is becoming increasingly difficult and confused as hospitals and universities collaborate under the multiple sponsorship. It can sell its services where appropriate. It can be staffed, in large part, by faculty whose career development in a conventional academic department or division is not interrupted. There is general recognition that no medical spokesman or biological or medical consultation is easily available to industry; the center should be expected to fill that role.

We suggest a single director (rather than co-directors representing engineering and biology) with a background in engineering or biological science rather than clinical medicine. We propose the center be built around a small administrative group, a small full-time staff of section chiefs and assistants, and a large number of part-time associates. A particular advantage of M.I.T.-Harvard association lies in the available numbers and variety of potential part-time associates. The gradual evolution of hybrid appointments might be anticipated, e.g., assistant professor of electrical engineering (engineering biology) or associate in medicine (engineering).

An important nonroutine administrative function will be the channeling of inquiries, particularly about potential collaborators of the availability of needed services. The importance of this function was repeatedly emphasized by members and consultants to the committee. Provisional, informal collaboration between engineers and biologists will continue, and here the center has a role to play as broker.

Three major divisions are suggested for the center, namely: services to bioscience, a section on human ecology, and a section on engineering applications in biology. The last would be the section most concerned with physiologic monitoring, physiologic measurement, and devices for therapy, and will be discussed separately. The ecology section would take for its field the application of systems engineering to both large and small biological and medical systems; questions of the economics and efficiencies of medical care delivery; and questions of interactions of large human and animal populations with their environments. The section on services to biosciences would include a minimum of an animal laboratory, routine shop facilities, a computer with consultative services, and a few carefully chosen special laboratories including biologic materials or preparations, as well as maintenance of specific cell lines and tissue culture, manufacture of high-cost, low-demand devices unsuitable for industrial development, the performance of tests or assays for which there is a continuing demand, and the important, currently needed standards laboratory for biologic measurements. Assay of prostaglandins is an example of a biochemical determination that is presently tedious, expensive, in demand, and greatly in need of either automated methods or new measurement concepts. This section requires an independent evaluation committee to determine the allocation of available resources between competing requests for services. It is expected that a close-working relationship with specialized advanced development laboratories, such as the Instrumentation Laboratory, would fill the roll of this section.

The engineering applications section, with its director and full-time assistant (probably graduate students), would maintain affiliations both with individuals in biological and medical sciences and with hospitals. This is the section most concerned with direct patient care, and it would be profitable to organize a team centered on each Harvard teaching hospital. Each of the hospitals maintain some type of clinical research unit, and patient contact would be most rewarding in that setting. Each hospital would have on its own staff an engineer working in medicine who would perform some investigative tasks and have a service function in the particular hospital. An association with the center would be rewarding for these individuals, who are often threatened with isolation from the main channel of engineering progress. The importance of bringing engineers concerned with medical matters into the life of the hospital cannot be overemphasized both for increased motivation and work satisfaction and increased qualitative understanding of the problems of hospital medicine.

The biological application section would maintain collaboration in the form of center associates in individual laboratories working with investigators in the biological sciences. Physiology is an obvious example but not the only one. The initial attraction would probably be the availability of fabrication capability, but we would hope that the attraction would eventually advance to the intellectual level rather than to the material level.

This section would, of course, also be concerned with therapeutic devices, a subject that ranges the whole distance from artificial internal organs to improvements in surgical instruments. The important areas in this field are similar to the second category of physiological monitoring problems in that important segments of the relevant basic science have not been studied sufficiently and also because development requires close and continuous collaboration between clinical scientists—in hospitals—and engineers.

Physiologic Monitoring and Measurement

Physiologic monitoring appears easily distinguishable from physiologic measurement. Monitoring we define as the first part of the process of treatment, in which information is gathered, processed, and evaluated, after which decisions are made and action taken.

Observation of the effects of therapy provides further information, used in turn to help decide the next action and modify the previous one. One of its purposes is to warn of impending changes. Part of this information can be conveniently acquired, processed, and recorded with electrical or mechanical devices; when these devices reach a certain level of complexity, data acquisition is called monitoring. It is, nevertheless, an extension of everyday medical procedures and not a substitute for them; and it follows that the responsibility for safety, adequacy, and utility of these methods is a part of primary patient responsibility. Applications in the other two parts of the therapeutic process—making decisions and taking action—hold promise for future development; and though they are usually sharply demarcated from monitoring, they should not be considered separate from it.

The assumptions, objectives, and methods of physiologic measurement are more familiar to most engineering scientists than are those employed in monitoring patients. One of the objectives is knowledge for its own sake. There is a fair degree of interaction between the two fields but an almost one-way flow of methods from physiologic measurement toward physiologic monitoring, although recently there has been a trend for novelties to originate in the clinical area rather than the physiology laboratory. Most evident in the field of physiologic measurement, but by no means peculiar to it, there is a strong inclination toward the do-it-yourself approach. Improvisation has real advantages and provides the competition to a more organized program of instrument development. There are positive values worthy of preservation in this cottage industry approach, one being its educational function. At the level of basic research, where close contact with the work and considerable study and reflection are essential, it may well be irreplaceable. An analogy is the use of certain hand methods in biochemical laboratories, even though automated methods or commercial laboratory services are available, primarily to instruct research personnel.

Generally speaking, monitoring methods in current use do not require large improvements in repeatability, accuracy, or precision. There is great need for improvements in safety, convenience, and cost. Current monitoring methods tend to be descriptive and seldom measure remaining reserve or the response to a perturbation.

Listed below are some examples of monitoring methods either now in use or on the horizon, with some remarks about their prospects for further development. Certain physical measurements are now made quite well, such as temperature, mass, electrical potential, pressure, and length. There are some problems, and for all of them, as mentioned before, there is room for improvements in cost, convenience, and safety. Developments in this category, however, could be pursued in a center isolated from a hospital; it is not easy to foresee important advantages here in the application of time, money, and talent.

A second category of physical measurement exists in which the objective can be defined, but present methods are unsatisfactory to achieve it. Improvements are needed at the conceptual level, the transducer level, and the interpretive level. Examples are volume and mass flow measurement of blood, air, biochemical substrate, and metabolic products, especially of a particular region or organ. Another example is acoustic measurements, now limited almost entirely to clinical auscultation, phonocardiography, and beginning work in ultrasonic scanning. Here much of the basic biological work remains to be done, and development can be expected to require parallel overlapping work in the animal laboratory, the engineering laboratory, and the hospital.

There is also a class of problems, generic rather than transducer or organ oriented, which deserves study, and which is suited to investigation by a center. This class concerns the interaction of a measuring device, particularly an implanted device, with the organism; attitudinal studies in connection with physiological monitoring; and evaluation of economic factors in monitoring. The growing problem of data reduction and utilization, particularly for long-term measurements, concerns all of the above.

Two specific examples have been considered in more detail. The first is recording and display of monitoring data presently considered useful without particular regard to development of new measurements. The second is recognition and treatment of respiratory failure, a compelling problem in present-day medicine.

Intensive Care Monitoring

The intensive care unit, in present-day practice, represents about 10 percent of a general hospital's total bed capacity. As a hospital facility, it may or may not include certain special care areas: coronary monitoring, respiratory, burn, or organ transplantation units.[1,2] Patients in an intensive care unit include the most critically ill of a hospital's patient population with the highest case fatality rate.

In a surgical intensive care unit, patients and their problems are not so uniform as in a respiratory unit or coronary monitoring area. Several groups of problems are nevertheless identifiable. These are:

1) Thermal burns.
2) Invasive sepsis: Shock due usually to blood stream infection from peritonitis or the urinary tract.

3) Shock due to hemorrhage, usually from the gastrointestinal tract.

4) Extensive trauma to multiple organ systems, most commonly due to automobile accident.

Although there are some common needs, each of these groups has different requirements for monitoring during the acute phase of the illness.

A number of problems in intensive care unit organization are seen as ripe for examination and innovation by engineering scientists. Some are architectural: a solution to the competing demands of easy observation and access, prevention of bacterial cross-contamination, and patient comfort has never been found. Some problems are organizational, and a major one is communication of data about patients to the often large number of people involved in their care. In particular, the quantity of simple physiologic information gathered and transcribed, usually by a nurse, is large and represents a considerable portion of the time she spends at the bedside, perhaps as much as 25 percent of it. These data are now tabulated on a single large sheet, which is soon covered with figures.

A further tabulation of this information is made for greater utility in clinical decision making. In a teaching hospital this is often the task of a senior medical student. Intake and output information is plotted cumulatively with results of laboratory determinations and physiological measurements. These so-called flow charts are quite different from patient to patient; one of the characteristics of the intensive care group, as mentioned, is variety.

There is a plain need for machine processing here. The desired outputs are:

1. Display of tabular and graphical information at the bedside, with capability for modification of the format.

2. A daily summary printout for the permanent record.

3. Special printouts generated through an on-line dialogue between machine and therapist to show correlations of events, therapy, and monitoring data appropriate to the particular patient.

Most inputs for this system exist or are obtainable in either analogue or machine-readable form. The standard physiologic transducers are compatible with the system. Laboratory data at Peter Bent Brigham Hospital is returned to the floor by teleprinter. Other inputs could be entered at a console.

This is a small-scale project that would make an immediate improvement in patient care. It should not be an effort to accumulate a large permanent file of undigested physiologic data, an approach that has not generally been useful. The byproducts offer an opportunity to study the monitoring process, to validate monitoring data against clinical events, to develop in-context display systems and methods for automatic control of sampling rates, and to establish the conceptual limitations of present notions of clinical monitoring.

Some beginnings have been made here and in Los Angeles, Alabama, and Salt Lake City, and other centers, but we suggest a somewhat different emphasis. The proposal is not for a hospital information system. Data handling rather than data collection is the objective and only then for a few intensive care patients where the data density is high.

This is an example of an enterprise requiring a mixed team of a systems analyst, a programmer, and an engineer experienced in interfacing and terminal design. It could be begun from a computer-rich position with gradual improvements in hardware economics: for example, analogue preprocessing of some of the data. First development might take place outside the hospital, but an early evaluation of a prototype device is required since the principal anticipated difficulties are in the human engineering rather than the transducer design, programming, or display.

RECOGNITION AND TREATMENT OF RESPIRATORY FAILURE

This is an example of a defined field with great opportunity for a programmed approach to clearly discernable objectives. The group of patients in question make an attractive choice for many of the same reasons that the larger intensive care group is an important one, e.g., most patients are without malignant or necessarily irreversible disease; there are demonstrable differences between results attainable with optimum care and with average care, optimum care, of course, requiring a considerably large expenditure of professional and semiprofessional time; and the basic science base on which clinical respiratory therapy is built, being pulmonary physiology, is a particularly mature division of organ physiology.

A problem engaging the attention of increasing numbers of people is that the prevalance of respiratory failure as a complication of other disease may be increasing; its incidence of recognition is certainly increasing. Evidence for awakening general interest is the recent NAS/NRC conference invoked at the request of the armed services to consider the problem of respiratory failure in military casualties.[3]

The following subdivisions of the problem suggest themselves:

1. A broad examination of dimensions including incidence and current solutions.

2. Methods for diagnosis and monitoring; the problems of the patient—transducer interface—are large here, and there is a need for new transducer development, e.g., impedance plethysmography.

3. Development of therapeutic devices, such as ventilators and oxygen therapy equipment and devices for long-term extracorporeal circulation in support of oxygenation.

The open question is whether the systems analysis approach is a useful one in this problem; it is by no means clear that this method has ever been able to fulfill its promise in application to medicine.[4] At the level of this report it is not possible to be more specific about project details. Further definition of opportunities could begin still another committee made up of a group to work in or supervise a program in respiratory failure.

[1] "The Intensive Care Unit," *Anesthesiology* 25 (1964) : 192.

[2] J. M. Kinney, "The Intensive Care Unit," *Bulletin of the American College of Surgeons* 51 (Sept.–Oct. 1966) : 201–204, 348–356.

[3] Conference on the Pulmonary Effects of Non-Thoracic Trauma, Washington, D.C., Feb. 29–Mar. 2, 1968.

[4] B. R. Smith, *The RAND Corporation* (Cambridge, Mass.: Harvard University Press, 1966).

MAY 23, 1968

Introductions and orientation included an apology for the loose definition of the committee's function. This is to extract from the presentations of the members and from the general discussion specific suggestions for organization of the most effective combination of resources of Harvard and M.I.T., particularly in the area of physiologic monitoring as a subdivision of biology and engineering. Initial discussion considered the several sorts of organization commonly proposed for this purpose, e.g.,

1. an institute of biomedical engineering;
2. a personnel directory service; and
3. a service facility: shop or laboratory.

Some objections appeared at this point. One was that game-playing and idea-collecting are too different from real planning to be of much help. Several members have found personal, informal consulting arrangements to be entirely satisfactory, and they questioned the need for a formal structure. It was also suggested that any consideration of how engineering sciences can be better applied in medicine and biology should be discussed as particular problems in biology, rather than in a framework of organizational ways and means.

Dr. Bernard Lown then reviewed the status of coronary monitoring. Briefly, coronary artery disease is now the cause of 25 percent of all sudden deaths. In 25 percent of these deaths, the fatal event is the first sign of the existence of coronary artery disease. Hospital mortality has been reduced by introducing coronary monitoring units. In them, myocardial irritability is recognized by counting ventricular premature beats and treatment with drugs or resuscitation by electrical defibrillation when necessary. A further reduction of any significance in hospital mortality from coronary artery disease cannot be expected, but the 70 percent rate of deaths that occur before admission should yield to a program of precoronary monitoring. Some gain is realizable from earlier admission or from the use of mobile resuscitation units, but their effects can be safely predicted to be small. Precoronary monitoring is based on the recognition that high-risk individuals can be described by age, personal history, family education, and screening facilities to monitor the large numbers of persons suspected of impending coronary occlusion, possibly with the help of pharmacologic or mechanical stress imposition to uncover latent myocardial electrical instability.

There are clearly defined instrumentation needs here:
1. A VBP counter.
2. Telemetry for EKG recording from the unencumbered patient.

For Dr. Lown, these needs are being met by collaboration with workers at Worcester Polytechnic Institute, initially in their consulting time and now with some grant support. This arrangement followed unsuccessful attempts to enlist help within the Harvard-M.I.T. staffs.

Discussion touched on several points. One was the recognized difficulty of persuading industry to undertake this sort of development. One of the reasons is funding, which is at present easier for academic departments than commercial firms; another is industry's problem in judging the quality of advice and requests from M.D.s. It was remarked that although the development of devices for specific well-defined functions of demonstrated utility might lack intellectual challenge, members with medical backgrounds are sometimes unable to predict what would be an interesting project to engineers. It was also noted that circumscribed problems are ideal for student or graduate projects.

The committee reconvened after visiting the Levine Cardiac Unit. Dr. Jere Mead reviewed the long history of pulmonary physiology at the Harvard School of Public Health. No outstanding measurement problems were seen to exist; existing transducers for flow, pressure, and volume are satisfactory and do not make heavy demands on current technology. Help with instrumentation is usually obtained on an ad hoc basis, and the results have been satisfactory to all concerned. An example is measurement of pulmonary ventilation by body surface movements: magnetometers were substituted for strings and pulleys after a coincidental conversation with an interested geophysicist.

Final discussion emphasized the marked difference between patient monitoring and physiologic measurement and acknowledged the tendency of engineers and biologists to underestimate the degree of empiricism in opposite fields and to overvalue self-taught skills in themselves.

JUNE 6, 1968

Dr. Bowditch described the Instrumentation Laboratory: it is one of the special laboratories of M.I.T., organizationally part of M.I.T.'s Division of Sponsored Research, has a staff of 2,000, and works mostly in aerospace guidance and control. To the visitor, several points stand out, chiefly its concept-to-hardware approach to problems, an enormous computation facility, a considerable variety of engineering sciences represented on the staff, and an obvious interest in undertaking small ad hoc instrument developments.

Three examples were presented:

1. The GDM viscosimeter, a development requested by Professor Edward Merrill and begun in 1961. It was recognized that existing viscosimeters were inappropriate for non-Newtonian biologic fluids (they required an impractically large sample and measured viscous forces at unphysiologically high shear rates) and an existing device, originally designed for another purpose, was adapted for measurement of the very small restoring forces required for biologic viscosimetry. Now synovial fluid and aqueous humor as well as blood and plasma are being studied. The GDM viscometer is an example of a device probably unsuited to commercial development because of small demand and high cost, but it is plainly of great utility. At the same time, it could not easily be built in the ordinary university shop. Consequently, several have been custommade.

2. A project in temperature biotelemetry was begun, again at an investigator's request and with the objectives fairly well defined by the nature of the project: study of circadian rhythms in rats. The problems have been very practical ones: antenna design, sealing implanted sensors, and elimination of interference from simultaneous use of several telemetry transmitters.

3. Another example is the adaptation of a scanning electron microscope to computer control for counting,

sizing, and perhaps identifying small particles (up to 2 microns in length). The immediate application is to air pollution studies but one aspect of the project is part of the larger problem of pattern recognition. The approach chosen has been to perform some logic functions in a special purpose interfacing device to reduce the size of the needed computer to something on the order of PDP-8.

Discussion brought out several points. One was that there is no easy way for the engineering developers of a device to evaluate its potential applications beyond those for which the development was originally requested. Obviously, this can never be more than guessed. The viscosimeter seems to be fully penetrating its field of potential application. Both biotelemetry and the scanning electron microscope have many promising, immediate applications; the problem is deciding which are ripe for development. The medical members were impressed by the degree of specialization in the engineering world and also by the accelerating rate of change in components and integrated circuit technology.

JUNE 28, 1968

The meeting began with a visit to the Massachusetts General Hospital's respiratory unit. The unit was established in 1961 for treatment of all types of respiratory failure. About two-thirds of the patients have been surgical cases (trauma, thoracic surgery, etc.). The overall mortality has been 228/598 or about 40 percent, but more significantly, uncomplicated ventilatory failure, exemplified by a series of patients with myasthenia gravis, has been treated without mortality. It was obvious during the visit that there is more care than monitoring concerned in treatment of these respirator patients and that the requirement for both attendance and supervision is greater than in most other types of clinical areas.

Dr. Bendixen discussed those measurements that have been found useful, to some extent for diagnosis, but largely as an aid in making decisions about treatment. They include simple volume measurements: vital capacity (or the volume that can be exhaled after a maximally deep breath), the maximum expiratory flow rate (self-explanatory), and a compliance measurement (the ratio of an inspired volume to the respirator pressure necessary to produce it). This last is recognized as a convenient clinical approximation only, because the pressure-volume characteristics of lung and chest wall is nonlinear. The arterial-alveolar partial pressure gradient of respiratory gases is measured, and a ratio of dead space volume (the part of lung volume not in equilibrium with pulmonary blood) to tidal volume (the volume of a single breath) is calculated.

It was pointed out that these measurements are made with simple tools—a water spirometer, flowmeter, and electrodes for blood gas tensions and pH; but even so, the idea that multiple measurements are necessary to describe a patient's status generates some resistance.

Discussion included the pros and cons of continuous measurement of those variables now measured intermittently, with agreement that as a principle this is desirable when feasible. Dr. Anliker emphasized the general advantage of working from a data-rich position in any enterprise involving signal analysis and the easier recognition of a singularity against as broad a background of contrasting signals as possible.

Dr. John Kinney was introduced, and he described the concepts that follow consideration of the human organism as an energy exchange device. One is that patients die because of some block in energy exchange and that the traditional observation of vital signs is really an attempt to observe one step in the process of energy transfer. A broader look at energy exchange is potentially useful. Input-output studies (e.g., measurement of gas exchange, intake of substrate, and heat loss) establish the limits within which the components of the human black box can be separated one from another. The examination of intermediary metabolism, particularly control of substrate utilization, should be as important in monitoring as measurement of pulmonary and circulatory factors in oxygen transport.

Dr. Kinney pointed out that in working in this field with engineers he has found that while they have an advantageous familiarity with network analysis, model making, and other mathematical tools required, it nonetheless takes about six months for a collaborating engineer to find his footing and work effectively and that first-hand, on-site experience is required.

The program for the meeting was as follows:
Introduction to the Massachusetts General Hospital Laboratory of Computer Science—Octo Barnett
Physiological Data Processing—Jim Poitras
Time-sharing system on JOSS—Neil Pappalardo
Patient Interviewing by Computer—Dave Swedlow
Automated Chemistry Laboratory—Peter Katona

Dr. Barnett kindly submitted to a long cross-examination about the computer's role in clinical medicine. He remains convinced that most of the possibilities foreseen for medical applications remain valid, but that early estimates of the time required for realization were wrong.

The Massachusetts General Hospital laboratory has an open-ended mandate to apply computer technology to hospital medicine, but the laboratory has elected not to become involved in direct patient monitoring. No analogue signals from patients are processed. It is believed that present-day patient monitoring is severely limited by the lack of correlation of analogue data with medical record information, and the objective has been to develop methods to get data from medical histories, X-ray reports, and laboratory results into a coordinated format for display and decision making.

The laboratory's association with M.I.T. has been rewarding. Almost all the staff has been found there, and through informal associations, there is access to a large pool of engineering competence.

This meeting, before and after dinner, was a less than completely successful attempt to get down to specific proposals, and for reasons listed in the main body of the report it was decided to emphasize the problem of recognition and treatment of respiratory failure.

There was general agreement that a study should begin with a broad examination of goals, emphasizing possible applications of newer systematic approaches to the decision-making process, and that this might be done first in around-the-table form.

A discussion of why monitoring systems fail reemphasized some of the previously discussed problems, e.g., clumsiness at the system-patient interface, lack of validation of information obtained, bad information processing, unfavorable economics, and infeasible laboratory techniques for bedside use.

The discussion ended with some speculation about the possible utility of the systems approach. Those who had some experience with practicioners of systems engineering were able to warn against expecting useful results from the methods without adequate description of the problem to which it is applied.

Individually Submitted Reports

EXTRACTS FROM A LETTER FROM DR. PETER KATONA

My main concern is as yet the lack of a somewhat deeper and more detailed examination of physiologic monitoring. In my view, monitoring involves to a very large extent the storage, retrieval, and reorganization of the collected data. No present system does even a halfway complete job (as far as I know), and these data-handling problems are probably as severe as the difficulties mentioned in the draft report. I think it is important to delve into some of the details of the monitoring problem (instrumentation, data collection, organization, etc.) and show where and why the center could really make a contribution. For example, many monitoring systems overburden their computer by sampling indiscriminately at a high rate. This collects a lot of data which manifests itself in filling up storage space and ends up doing relatively little for the patient. Analogue preprocessing of data seems very much ignored. Easy and within-context display of the data is another important challenge.

We probably should provide the steering committee with more proposals that are specific to physiological monitoring. For example, one question is the testing of whatever monitoring system the center develops. Should the center have a clinical unit, or should it collaborate with one or more of the local hospitals? (Most other panels tend to favor the latter approach; this certainly seems more practical to me.) It would also be helpful to set up some priorities; would the center tackle all aspects of monitoring right away, or develop the system piecemeal? I don't know the answer, but my personal interest starts at the output-signal of the transducer. Also, giving a very rough idea of a budget may be appropriate.

EXTRACTS FROM A REPORT SUBMITTED BY
DR. EDWARD BURGER

To some extent it undoubtedly is true that the current desire to monitor physiological function and well being of a man as a part of a "system" within a spacecraft has encouraged diversification and generalization of the trend toward use of technology in health care. Although this desire to make objective measurements by electronic or mechanical means may have been accelerated by the space effort, the trend would probably have existed anyway.

The term "patient monitoring" is characteristically associated with the measurement of physiological function in the acutely ill patient. Typically most articles written about monitoring discuss methods and systems used in coronary care units and operating rooms. A proper perspective would assign a broader set of tasks to monitoring. I submit that the following all represent current situations where objective measurements are useful for the diagnostic or therapeutic decision-making process.

1. *Alerting to the occurrances of abrupt or significant changes in function in the acutely ill.* This is useful in the immediate situation only if the changes measured are valid, if their mechanism or relation to a state of health is understood, and if an appropriate intervention is possible.

2. *Assistance in recognition of improbable but important events among patients who may be unwell but not necessarily acutely unwell.* The rationale in this case is really the most efficient and productive use of existing health-care resources (people, time, money, and things). That is, this represents an example of the introduction of technology in order to conserve human resources or make them more efficient. Specific examples might include patients in nursing homes, other custodial care situations, or poorly manned wards. Again, however, the measurement must be an appropriate one and intervention must be possible in order to make the measurement useful.

3. *Diagnostic monitoring*. Provocative tests such as the exercise EKG are examples. The demonstration of infrequent changes in function or abnormalities is typically the aim. There is an additional related field: the development of objective instruments to assist in the performance of the classical physical examination. Required here is the evolution of transducers to make more objective some of the manipulations practiced in palpation and percussion.

Inventories similar to the above can be found in articles on this subject (Wolff, 1966). Some generalities have been made about patient monitoring that are worth repeating:

1. Patient monitoring, as have other types of objective measurements made on patients, has suffered a long legacy of uncertain support from the members of the medical profession. Soma Weiss wrote in 1941:

"In recent years, in contrast to the past, few books have been written on symptoms. Beginning with the end of the nineteenth century, the interest in the pathogenesis of disease and the use of laboratory methods led to an underestimation of the value of the interpretation of symptoms. Indeed, many still consider a good history and a proper evaluation of complaints to be less important today than in the past. This is, however, a serious misconception.

"A good physician is one who uses the least number of laboratory procedures to arrive at the correct conclusion. Nowadays, putting the patient through the mill is not infrequently confused with thoroughness. . . .

"Before the advent of modern clinical investigation, symptoms were for the most part correlated with the findings of the physical examination and eventually with the morphologic changes observed at postmortem. The fundamental nature of symptoms could not be studied because of the lack of objective methods sufficiently sensitive for such study. Hence, the symptoms of each disease were often analyzed empirically. With the discovery in recent years of new chemical, physical, and physiological methods, has come the first study of the fundamental mechanism of many symptoms such as dyspnea, orthopnea, cyanosis, nausea, vomiting, unconsciousness, and pain. If we understand the physiology of cyanosis, we can at once evaluate its possible significance. And so we find the interpretation of symptoms on a firmer foundation today than ever before.

"The fact that complicated instruments are essential to the fundamental study of a symptom does not mean that the physician in his daily practice must necessarily use these instruments. Once investigation has established the significance of a clinical phenomenon, the intelligent use of the conclusion reached suffices in the practice of medicine." (Weiss in Meakins, 1941)

This represents a traditional, relatively conservative attitude toward the art and mechanics of the practice of medicine and there are good reasons for it.

"When a patient presents himself or herself before the medical man, that patient is commonly a stranger. . . . How, then, must the young practitioner commence his examination? Some fly at the patient with a stethoscope, or call in the aid of divers instruments of precision. These latter are not to be ignored, certainly; but there is much to be done besides resorting to these valuable aids. Instruments of precision come in more fittingly at the close of the examination rather than at the beginning!"

However, this point of view deserves periodic reexamination. Machinery for rapid, inexpensive, and accurate mass chemical analysis of small blood samples has begun to force a change in attitudes toward the proper utility of laboratory procedures. Perhaps one of the most extreme examples is seen in the concept of the multiphasic screening clinic. There may be some parallels that can be drawn between the laboratory diagnostic methods and electronically instrumented measurements here described as monitoring methods.

Relative to most physical systems, measurement of function in the human system is a very gross and superficial affair. This is undoubtedly more true in the clinical situation than in the research laboratory. There are perhaps two major reasons for this. There often exists uncertainty about what to measure because of imperfect understanding of the mechanism of physiology and the disease processes. This is additionally reflected in the inability of the clinician to describe adequately to his engineering counterpart what it is he wants to sample by way of an instrument. Secondly, although the clinician is generally confined to "nondestructive" testing of his patient, his abilities to make manifest what is beneath the surface of the integument are severely limited. Accordingly, the measurements that are commonly made on patients are typically indirect and chosen at least partly because they are accessible or easy to perform (temperature, pulse, and respiration, for example).

"The temperature *chart* may be considered the barometer of the patient's condition. It is one of the few means of accurate observation that we have at our disposal, and should never be neglected. Some surgeons of wide experience will sometimes studiously ignore the chart and pass their judgment of a patient's condition upon his general aspect, his posture, the appearance of his tongue, and all these aided by intuition. Their deductions may often appear brilliant, but their example is a dangerous one for the younger man to follow." (Crandon, L. R. G., 1911)

This practice of measuring functions that are accessible and that are traditional to measure continues to the present. Patient monitoring systems usually display temperature, blood pressure, respiration, and EKG signals. These represent the bulk of the continuous measurements made on astronauts in flight (National Aeronautics and Space Administration, 1966). By contrast, it seems very likely that other measurements more related to mechanisms of disease and complications would be appropriate if monitoring systems are to fulfill a real purpose.

The term "physiological measurement" is used to designate the concept of the sampling of physiological function in the physiological research laboratory as opposed to the clinical setting. In fact, the distinction (as in the case of applied versus basic research) is not clear-cut, and there is much overlapping. However, there are certain generalities that may be made to characterize physiological measurement.

Typically, a high degree of accuracy and resolution is demanded in physiological research and is simply a reflection of the rigorousness of the research effort. Measurement is the major goal, not treatment and rehabilitation. Accuracy accrues from a combination of superior equipment and careful operation of it. A sizable amount of research, time, and effort is expended on the development of transducers and associated conditioning and recording equipment. Much of this effort is carried on personally by the experimenter.

The physiological experimenter will commonly accept bread boarding; convenience, size, and arrangement are not of great importance. He may not be unhappy about having to analyze his results in order to interpret them. The clinician, by contrast, is generally unhappy about any inconveniences in the design and operation of equipment. Accordingly, he would strongly prefer the most convenient display of the data possible so they would be immediately meaningful to him. To him, data reduction may be a problem.

It is traditionally a common practice for a basic researcher to develop and build a large part of the equipment which he employs. Measuring equipment is no exception. This practice comes about for a variety of reasons, and there are a number of undoubted advantages to commend it. Often there is nothing available commercially to satisfy the researcher's needs. Or, although commercial devices might be available, they may not perform satisfactorily for his purposes. By designing his own piece of equipment, the experimenter may be able to increase his confidence in the data he gathers. This is consonant with his habit of maintaining close personal control over all parts of the experimental enterprise. It has been traditional to be generally resourceful in the research laboratory. Even with the trend toward institutionalization of research in latter years, individual or small-team efforts toward research remain the commonest practice. This type of approach has a number of advantages, but at the same time there are inefficiencies in this practice. That is, to some varying extent, the biological investigator who devotes his own exclusive energies to the development of mechanical and electrical measuring devices may be doing himself a disservice if that task could be done as well and faster in concert with an engineer or physicist.

References

L. R. G. Grandon, *Surgical After-Treatment* (Philadelphia: W. B. Saunders Co., 1911).

J. M. Fothergill, *The Physiological Factor in Diagnosis* (New York: William Wood & Co., 1884).

Meakins, J. C.: *Symptoms in Diagnosis* (Boston: Little, Brown, and Company, 1941).

National Aeronautics and Space Administration, Gemini Midprogram Conference Including Experimental Results, NASA Manned Spacecraft Center, Houston, Texas, 1966.

H. Wolff, "The Monitron Project," *Journal of Advances in Medical Instrumentation* 1, no. 2 (1966): 22–27.

Task Group Report on Physiological Systems Analysis

Laurence R. Young
ASSOCIATE PROFESSOR OF AERONAUTICS
MASSACHUSETTS INSTITUTE OF TECHNOLOGY, CHAIRMAN

Lawrence B. Evans
ASSISTANT PROFESSOR OF CHEMICAL ENGINEERING
MASSACHUSETTS INSTITUTE OF TECHNOLOGY

William R. Ferrell
ASSISTANT PROFESSOR OF MECHANICAL ENGINEERING
MASSACHUSETTS INSTITUTE OF TECHNOLOGY

Stephen J. Fricker
DEPARTMENT OF OPHTHALMOLOGY
MASSACHUSETTS EYE AND EAR INFIRMARY

James C. Houk
DEPARTMENT OF PHYSIOLOGY
HARVARD MEDICAL SCHOOL

Howard T. Hermann
PSYCHIATRIST
NEUROPHYSIOLOGY LABORATORY
McLEAN HOSPITAL

Peter G. Katona
ASSISTANT PROFESSOR OF ELECTRICAL ENGINEERING
MASSACHUSETTS INSTITUTE OF TECHNOLOGY

Robert J. McLaughlin
LECTURER ON SYSTEMS ANALYSIS
HARVARD UNIVERSITY

Jacob L. Meiry
ASSISTANT PROFESSOR OF AERONAUTICS
MASSACHUSETTS INSTITUTE OF TECHNOLOGY

Douglas R. Waud
ASSISTANT PROFESSOR OF PHARMACOLOGY
HARVARD MEDICAL SCHOOL

Alfred D. Weiss
ASSISTANT IN NEUROLOGY
MASSACHUSETTS GENERAL HOSPITAL

David M. Worthen
DEPARTMENT OF OPHTHALMOLOGY
MASSACHUSETTS EYE AND EAR INFIRMARY

Summary

Although the current level of interdisciplinary research in physiological systems analysis is quite high in the Boston area, the road to collaborative research is difficult, and a number of specific important research projects are either delayed or never begun. The need for continual, fruitful interaction between physical scientists and life scientists, availability and staffing of engineering facilities and hospital services, and formal and informal educational resources for students and the visibility and attractiveness of these activities would all be greatly enhanced by a bioengineering center. For the purposes of our activities, the center should be located on the M.I.T. campus; its major clinical facilities should be in the form of two research wards and associated engineering laboratories in the hospitals. The center will require substantial participation by physiologists and physicians, some full-time and some part-time, as well as by engineers. Preferably, the administration would be carried out jointly by M.I.T. and Harvard. In addition to the faculty, graduate students, and postdoctoral researchers, the need for a nucleus of staff engineers and medical technicians is stressed. Nine major projects in physiological systems analysis are outlined, many of them extensions or continuations of ongoing projects at M.I.T. or Harvard; approximately sixty people using some twenty-five laboratory rooms would be involved. Among the facilities considered essential are satellite and central computer services, animal facilities and laboratories, an environmental test chamber, a vehicle simulator, an optics laboratory, an instrument room, an electronic shop, a histology laboratory, use of an electron microscope, machine shop and model shop, a medical examining room, minimum local facilities for patient care, a photolab, and appropriate document and publication staffs.

Introduction: Envisaged Collaboration in Physiological Systems Analysis

Physiological systems analysis entails the application of applied mathematics or engineering technology to the analysis of some living system. By its nature it requires specialized knowledge of the biological system under study, as well as broad background in the mathematical techniques available for analyzing the system or for designing critical experiments. Although Cannon's *Wisdom of the Body* was published in the early thirties, most of the quantitative modeling of complex physiological systems has taken place in the last fifteen years, usually through genuine collaboration between engineers and physiologists, at least in defining the problems. Because of the vertical structure of engineering education, most physiologists are not equipped to apply appropriate analysis with confidence. Engineers, on the other hand, in addition to requiring the specialized knowledge of the system they are modeling, also need the close cooperation of life scientists to prevent them from modeling systems that are unrelated to physiological reality. Where possible, they need guidance to orient the modeling effort toward diagnostic applications. (A frequently heard criticism of models of complex biological systems is the absence of reality in the engineering approximations.) Closer collaborative efforts among engineers and physicians are necessary to further the development of biological control modeling and speed its application towards patient care. In most cases, ad hoc research efforts in this area involve consultation between the medical and engineering schools rather than a true collaboration. We feel that this situation would be alleviated by a center in which both life scientists and engineers were present in large enough numbers to maintain continual interaction and equality of standing.

In the specific area of physiological systems analysis, the committee feels that the most important interactions are among people who are working on the same problem (e.g., cardiovascular or neuromuscular) from different viewpoints, rather than among people who are using the same viewpoint (e.g., computer simulation) on a variety of different biological problems. Applied mathematicians in general want closer contact with life science people doing research on the same problems they themselves are interested in, rather than increased contact with other mathematicians or engineers.

The subcommittee participants were deliberately chosen from different areas of M.I.T. and Harvard and asked to report on the relevant research programs in their departments. Written reports, appended to this report, include summaries of current research projects, the research programs projected for the next five to ten years, and the facility requirements associated with these programs. A wide variety of these projects were discussed, and those nine that appear most appropriate for a bioengineering center and would seem to gain most from the resulting collaborative efforts are listed here:

1. Models of ventricular action. The dynamics of ventricular function may be modeled mathematically, and the model may be checked with experiments to yield a better understanding of the manner in which the ventricle operates. The introduction of mathematical notions yields a conceptual framework describing cardiac muscle operation that may be of direct clinical interest in understanding the nature of a diseased heart and evaluating the quality of the muscle involved. By using combinations of conventional models for individual muscle elements to yield a distribution of properties in the ventricular configuration, one can calculate pressure as a function of time and evaluate the pressure-flow impedance dynamics for cardiac muscle. This research reflects the interests of investigators at the department of applied mathematics and department of physiology at Harvard and at the Peter Bent Brigham Hospital.

2. Cardiovascular control system modeling. Study of the cardiovascular control system has for many years been of prime interest in this field. Some of the specific topics to be considered for current study include the following: blood pressure regulation system and the carotid sinus reflex, and consideration of the entire cardiovascular control loop as a multioutput system. The three primary outputs to be modeled are actions of the automatic nerve system on the heart, actions on the peripheral resistance, and actions on the capacitance vessels, both in the steady state and during transient responses. In addition, the roles played by pressure receptors at various points in the cardiovascular system

is to be studied. Our past work in this area has been chiefly in the department of electrical engineering and the Reserch Laboratory of Electronics in collaboration with the Massachusetts General Hospital. There is also interest in this research at the Harvard Department of Physiology.

3. Postural control. The interaction of the various orientation sensors, especially the visual and vestibular organs, on man's postural control is considered a problem particularly appropriate for a bioengineering center and is in the mainstream of interest of at least two groups. In brief, the modeling of the vestibular system must be augmented by further consideration of the neurophysiology at the peripheral end and the neuromuscular action involved in postural control. The role of the cerebellum in particular has been underestimated in the past, and although there is already collaboration in this area, it is felt that a joint effort on the neurophysiology of the postural control system would help in making more accurate localizations of neurophysiological damage. In addition to health care and the benefits and contributions to basic understanding, postural control efforts have such nondiagnostic applications as actively controlled prostheses or space or underwater exploration suits. It is also directly applicable to the man-machine systems problems of vehicle control.

4. Total sensory-motor systems, including man-machine systems and attention. This omnibus research category includes a number of topics associated with higher level human processing and specifically includes manual control, the motor effector side of brain function, and cognitive processes as related to direction of attention, decision-making, and detection theory. The investigation of how we focus visual attention is crucial in understanding learning. The physiological correlations of attention shifting are to be investigated, as well as the behavioral aspects. The relation of visual attention to eye movements continues to be of interest. The motor effector discharge pattern represents a fruitful area for analytic modeling using the techniques of decomposing complex motor movement into sequences of elementary programmed patterns, and an experimental psychologist and a neurophysiologist are attacking this problem. A

crucial question that can be answered by such collaborative efforts is the role of the cerebellum in motor effector loops. The current level of understanding of electrophysiology and technology for investigating the cerebellum in new ways to unravel its electroanatomical connections promises to disclose the operation and function of some of its circuitry in terms of what it does for the body. Manual control modeling and improvements in man-machine interfaces represent a significant on-going effort in the M.I.T. mechanical engineering department.

The applications of this research to practical engineering problems are obvious. In addition, the direct or indirect benefits of such research in the areas of artificial intelligence and pattern recognition must be recognized.

5. Transduction and information processing in the nervous system. In many cases, information processing is limited by the capabilities of the sense organ, which can no longer transduce information given to it so that it can be further processed. A fruitful project for collaborative research among an engineer, a neurophysiologist, and a psychologist would be to investigate forms in which the nervous system can accept information and, similarly, manners in which physical information can be transduced. (Efforts in information transmission through the tactile sense, unfortunately, ran into many serious problems.) The kinds of transduction necessary might involve changing the form of input energy, or filtering in a general sense, including transformations on the frequency spectrum. There is clearly a link between the efforts suggested and the goals of the task group on sensory aims. Interest has been expressed in this area at the Massachusetts Eye and Ear Infirmary.

6. Modeling the respiratory control system. Mathematical models and computer simulations for the regulation of the respiratory system have been built up to enormously complicated general purpose computer models with large numbers of unknown parameters. There have been notable successes in using the model to explain physiological phenomena, in particular Cheyne-Stokes breathing. Significant research possibilities exist in developing detailed limited purpose models to represent particular respiratory phenomena or dis-

eases. The research will be carried out jointly by a mathematician familiar with modeling biological systems and a respiratory physiologist. Modeling of the ventilation-perfusion ratio and the operation of the lung also shows some promise. Associated research would be carried out on mechanical properties of lungs, again joining the talents of a physiologist and someone in applied mechanics.

7. Intraocular pressure modeling. The significant clinical problems of glaucoma and the importance of early detection emphasize the relevance of a basic study of regulation of intraocular pressure. Specific questions concern the degree of active or passive regulation of pressure via in-flow or out-flow of vitreous humor, the effect of changes in the vessels, the significance of facility (1/resistance) and pseudofacility, and the relevance of changes in scleral rigidity. Development of mathematical models carried out in close conjunction with studies of normal and diseased eyes would hopefully yield a significant index for parameters that would be more useful clinically than those currently measured. Work has previously been done in the department of aeronautics and astronautics, and collaboration from the Massachusetts Eye and Ear Infirmary seems assured.

8. Regulation of body fluid volume and composition. This is a complex biological control problem which has received very little modeling effort. Some current work on the osmoregulatory system is being carried out at the Harvard department of physiology, and interesting modeling of kidney function has been a joint research project between members of the Harvard department of applied mathematics and of the Tufts New England Medical Center. In this area, interest is high, and the beneficial effects of collaborative research are evident.

9. Models of drug effects. The dynamics of the uptake and distribution of drugs may be treated through compartmental analysis and analyzed to increase understanding of a number of pharmacological problems. At present the mathematical approaches used are quite straightforward, and the type of pharmacological research currently being done in the Harvard Medical School, while appropriate to a bioengineering center, can also be carried out in the present context.

Criteria for Ranking the Proposed Physiological Systems Analysis Projects

Six criteria were considered relevant to the evaluation of the proposed projects, and each criterion was quantified into three possible levels. The results are shown in Table 1, in which a plus indicates maximal ranking, a zero an intermediate level, and a minus a minimum. Notice that in the first and fourth columns, all projects have pluses: the first column represents the contribution to basic understanding, and it is characteristic of all the projects on physiological systems analysis that they are research-oriented with goals of increasing our understanding of the function of biological systems. Those projects that were discussed but not deemed sufficiently appropriate to a bioengineering center are not included, which explains the uniform ranking in column four. Column two is the contribution to health care rates : a plus ranking represents a rather direct application in the forseeable future, affecting diagnosis, instrumentation, or treatment; a zero represents some possible future direct application of uncertain nature; and a minus indicates that although the project is in the health sciences, it is primarily of a basic research nature. The rankings in column 3 represent the project's possible contributions to nonmedical applications, including such bioengineering oriented activities as bionics, man-vehicle interaction, and artificial intelligence for pattern recognition. The availability of resources indicated in column 5 refers primarily to the existence on the current staffs of M.I.T. or Harvard of senior research people committed to investigations in subject areas as well as facilities. A plus indicates that both the medical and engineering faculty members are currently in Boston and working separately or together on these problems; a zero indicates either that one of the other faculty members must be brought in to work on the problem or that there is a shortage of facilities; the minus in column 5 relating to drug action indicates the presumed likelihood of continuing this project outside the proposed center.

Table 1: Physiological Systems Analysis Projects

Project	Basic Research	Health Care	Nonmed. Contrib.	Appropriate for Center	Availability of Resources	Cost [a]	Number of Lab Rooms
Ventricle model	+	0	−	+	+	0	1
CV system model	+	0	−	+	0	+	3
Postural model	+	+	+	+	+	+	6
Transduction and information processing	+	0	+	+	+	+	9
Sensory-Cognitive-Effector models (man-machine)	+	−	0	+	0	0	1
Respiratory model	+	−	−	+	0	0	1
Intraocular pressure	+	+	−	+	0	0	1
Body fluid volume and composition	+	0	−	+	+	0	2
Drug action model	+	+	−	+	−	0	2

[a] Cost: + = Annual budget > $150,000
0 = Annual budget > $50,000

Administration of a Bioengineering Center

The committee on physiological systems analysis felt that although a variety of administrative forms could be used for a bioengineering center, it would find it most advantageous to have a center administered jointly by Harvard and M.I.T. It seems clear that, since for the projects mentioned a significant contribution comes from Harvard Medical School as well as considerable interest at Harvard's division of engineering and applied physics, joint administration is appropriate. The likelihood of faculty members from Harvard spending periods of full-time research or continuing on an extensive part-time basis at the bioengineering center and the feasibility of having Harvard students do their research in a bioengineering center would both be enhanced by joint administration. A relevant consideration for both the M.I.T. and Harvard participants was that research at the center would not be considered a step away from the home department. Transfer of equipment currently being used in the two schools might be facilitated through a jointly administered center.

A steering committee of senior engineers and physicians to review projects and disperse seed research money would be exceedingly desirable and would give a measure of recognition to younger researchers in the center.

Location

Since all of the projects involve engineering, and since not all of the activities of the bioengineering center are related directly to patient care, the physiological systems analysis committee recommends locating the proposed center on the M.I.T. campus. Nevertheless, it recognizes the importance of contact with patients for motivation and the proper definition of problems. For our purposes, only a few beds will be necessary in or near the bioengineering center, although medical examining rooms would be desirable. Primary contact with patients would take place in two research wards, with associated engineering laboratories located at the Massachusetts General Hospital and in the Harvard Medical

School area. Each ward would have an associated engineering laboratory outpost of the center. The engineering laboratories in the hospital outpost would have a small full-time engineering and technician staff and would serve as a home for engineering faculty and students in the hospital. The center should provide ample space and facilities for medical colleagues who spend only part of their time on this research activity.

Staffing

While recognizing the desirability of maintaining a high proportion of faculty and students in the bioengineering center, the committee also feels that a strong, full-time engineering and support staff is necessary to make contributions to health care and carry ideas beyond the thesis level. Engineering students working unsupervised in a hospital can create a burden. Some of this full-time staff should be located in the hospital outposts of the center and most of it in the bioengineering center itself. At the research investigator level, the primary requirements of the physiological systems analysis group seems to be for additional help in physiology. In particular, at least two full-time physiologists should be added to the staff to work on the cardiovascular and respiratory projects. The vast number of techniques to be mastered in some of the experimental physiological fields makes it essential that experienced biomedical technicians be available to help students and initiate engineers into the complexities of biological systems.

Facilities

This task group feels the need for a number of facilities in a proposed bioengineering center, many of which could be shared with other groups participating, and some of which are currently available at M.I.T. or Harvard.

1. Computation. Nearly all of the modeling projects involve computation for data processing or simulation of a biological system. In addition, many of these projects use special purpose computers for on-line data taking during experiments. For the proposed research projects, the investigators need a number of small (approxi-

mately 8K memory) dedicated digital computers in the laboratories and priority time-sharing access to a large central computer. The ideal central computer would have terminals in several animal laboratories, each terminal possessing A-D and D-A conversion and a graphics display. A number of small analog computers are useful for training graduate students in this area and would save tying up a larger machine. Most of the researchers felt the desirability of access to a large, versatile, hybrid computer for their modeling work. Extensions to the hybrid computer currently in the man-vehicle laboratory might be appropriate for some of the modeling efforts.

2. Animal facilities. Most of the proposed projects will involve constant interplay between mathematical modeling and the physiological system, and the desirability of having animal laboratories in the center is clear. Animals smaller than primates would suffice. At least two laboratories for doing animal surgery and keeping chronic preparations are required. Sharing animal laboratories while experiments are in progress seems unrealistic.

3. Pathology and histology laboratories with appropriate staffs.

4. A general medical facility that can be used to examine patients brought into the center.

5. An environmental test chamber with facilities for controlling atmospheric constituents, pressure, and other environmental variables.

6. A general purpose, moving base, vehicle simulator. Such a simulator, providing motion cues and simulated visual surroundings is necessary for studies of postural control, the motor effector system, and several man-machine problems.

8. The following engineering facilities, to be shared by all the researchers in the center, are extremely desirable:

a. a machine shop, properly staffed, to produce prototype equipment and a model shop where students can work;

b. an optics laboratory;

c. an instrument room that stocks, circulates, and services electronic and mechanical instruments; and

d. an electronics laboratory staffed by a design engineer

and technicians capable of taking on the straightforward electronics design problems associated with any laboratory activity.

9. General facilities. Desirable services would be a technical publications department and documentation specialists available to all researchers in the center, a specialized reading room that would concentrate on current literature and subliterature, and a seminar room.

10. Clinical facilities. As mentioned above, the proper clinical facilities would be located primarily in at least two research wards at the hospitals, devoted exclusively to projects of the bioengineering center.

Education

We recognize that for many years to come most of the research in bioengineering will be conducted by people trained principally in the life sciences or engineering, but not in both. Consequently, educational activities associated with the center are extremely important. Most of the education will continue to take place in the research laboratories through informal daily contact among students and faculty. In addition, however, because of many of the common requirements, at least two courses should be introduced.

A basic course in some engineering concepts should be made available to the biologists and medical personnel (at either the pre- or postdoctoral level) at the center to work on physiological systems analysis. We envision a specially tailored one-semester or preferably a one-year course that would include: computer structures and programming; the beginnings of numerical analysis; difference equations through partial differential equations; and sufficient introduction to complex variables to be able to recognize transfer functions and Laplace transforms. Additionally, either as part of this introductory course or as a separate offering, we recommend a short course in biostatistics.

Educational gaps among engineers working in this area are less easily filled because of the variety of physiological systems they may be working on. Taking as our model the master's degree student or the student beginning a doctoral program, we recommend offering him a one-year course in general physiology, emphasizing systems aspects. Although a full semester in cellular physiology is not required, the course should begin with an introduction to the study of physiology, followed by some consideration of cellular physiology and pathophysiology, and review the normal physiology of the organs. It should prepare the students for advanced courses or further reading in any of the medical specialties. An important adjunct to the general physiology course is a physiology laboratory for all the engineers. Advanced electives in bioengineering would presumably be among those available at Harvard Medical School. We also strongly recommend an interchange between medical students and engineering students, who should be brought into the hospital environment frequently.

Research Activities of Group Members

PROFESSOR LAWRENCE B. EVANS, M.I.T.

Work in the area of physiological systems analysis is a logical extension of the type of work done by the chemical engineer in conventional chemical process systems analysis. The chemical engineer is interested primarily in physiological systems in which a chemical processing function is an essential part. Examples include the artificial kidney, blood oxygenators, life-support systems for astronautics, and aquanautics. The techniques used in modeling, design, simulation, optimization, and control of chemical processes can also be applied to chemical processing systems in which a living organism is an essential element.

WORK NOW BEING DONE

Professors E. W. Merrill, K. A. Smith, and L. B. Evans have been active in investigating the engineering problems associated with the artificial kidney and the artificial lung. This work has been done with the collaboration of Drs. E. W. Salzman, W. G. Austen, and G. Baker, all of the Massachusetts General Hospital and Professor G. L. Brownell of the nuclear engineering department. Mr. Clark K. Colton, working under their direction, has developed a new technique for the determination of membrane permeability. The data thus generated are being applied in a study of the behavior of a single module of an artificial kidney. Mr. A. N. Dravid is now undertaking a study of mass transfer in helical coils for possible use in the artificial kidney. By virtue of the induced secondary flow, a helical coil presents less tube-side resistance to transfer than does the corresponding straight tube. This, then, could lead to artificial lungs and kidneys considerably more compact than those used at present.

A doctoral thesis project by Mr. Robert Havlin, under the supervision of Professors E. R. Gilliland and L. B. Evans, has been directed toward development for environmental control of a simple system to remove from the atmosphere acidic gases such as carbon dioxide, a system that can be regenerated electrically without direct application of heat. Such a system would be useful in a zero-gravity spacecraft environment.

Professor R. C. Reid has directed research into the engineering problems associated with life support systems for astronautics and aquanautics. The goal of this work is the design and optimization of such a system on the basis of cost, weight, volume, and reliability.

FUTURE WORK

Over the next three to five years, there will be a continuation and gradual expansion of present work. Some of the work presently being done by Professor L. B. Evans on control of conventional chemical processes will probably be extended to include control of physiological systems that function as a chemical process.

FACILITIES NEEDED

A reasonable level of activities for the chemical engineering department in this area might include the following:
four to five faculty members each devoting about 25–30 percent of their time to research supervision
four to six full-time research assistants involved in doctoral thesis investigations
five to ten half-time research assistants at the M.S. level
one or two full-time professionals

The facilities would include: office space, bench-scale laboratory space, and access to a large-scale digital computer (such as the IBM 360/65) on either a batch or time-sharing basis. Each thesis research project usually involves construction of specialized apparatus in the area of $2,000 to $6,000 and requires instruments for measuring and recording such process variables as temperature, pressure, flow rate, and chemical composition.

T. B. SHERIDAN, W. R. FERRELL, D. E. WHITNEY, M.I.T.

A. CURRENT RESEARCH RELATED TO HUMAN OPERATOR MODELING

1. Remote Manipulation supervised or directly controlled by an operator: strategies for dealing with delay and lag and the use of verbal language for commanding subtasks and interacting with a semiautonomous manipulator. A parallel aspect of the work is development of schemes for implementing the remote device's ability to achieve subgoals on its own.

2. Controls and displays: modeling switching behavior for various displays for time-optimal control of second-order systems; and the use of preview in control tasks, information transmission tasks, and maze solving.

3. Decision making and information processing in manual control: ability of a controller to predict the success of a maneuver from the circumstances and decide whether or not to try it; and transient effects of sudden changes in information load as related to taking over control from dual mode system.

4. Physiological: Models of the dynamics of the arm in rapid positioning with accuracy; and of the structure of the lateral geniculate nucleus in visual intensity discrimination.

B. ANTICIPATED DIRECTIONS FOR FUTURE WORK

It is likely that in the future there will be even greater emphasis on manipulation, decision making, and tasks involving cognitive information processing rather than on traditional tracking and control models. It is expected that in connection with manipulation, remote medical treatment and diagnosis will receive greater attention and that prototype systems will be put to test. The general question of supervision of and communication with sophisticated machines that can solve problems and make decisions is of interest. So, too, are questions related to interaction among people in systems, e.g., in traffic.

Improved facilities of three kinds will be needed for experimental work: manipulator hardware, simulation and display equipment, and expanded on-line computer capability. These facilities are necessary to simulate the complex systems implied by supervisory control and to meet the increased data-taking and processing requirements of experiments in which the subjects' behavior is relatively unconstrained and the number of possible options and strategies is relatively large.

DR. STEPHEN J. FRICKER

I. CURRENT PROJECTS

A. Clinical investigation of light-induced retinal and occipital potentials. This involves measurement of the amplitude and phase of signals at varying frequencies, and the system is designed to operate with clinical patients.

B. Measurement of eye position, velocity, and acceleration. The system is not yet in clinical use but is being designed to handle clinical material in place of trained personnel.

C. Application of computer technology to large-scale data storage and retrieval. Immediate application of this is possible at the pathology laboratory at the Massachusetts Eye and Ear Infirmary. A much larger scale undertaking is envisaged with the vision information center.

II. PROJECTS FOR THE NEXT FIVE YEARS

A. A continuation of the present projects. The extent of this would depend upon the availability of money, space, and personnel.

B. If we can obtain reasonable computer facilities, I think there will be a large expansion of investigation involving their use. Some of our analog devices undoubtedly would be changed, and more ambitious signal processing matters could be undertaken.

C. Again depending upon the availability of computer facilities, it is apparent that there would be considerable scope for the application of computer methods in running a hospital ward. It is not clear how much we might be engaged in this, particularly as the Massachusetts General Hospital is active in the field, but undoubtedly there would be problems peculiar to our own institution.

III. DESIRABLE FACILITIES

These may be listed very simply as:
A. Space
B. People
C. Money

At present there is literally no unused space at the Massachusetts Eye and Ear Infirmary. There are active plans, however, for building a new hospital facility, in which we may be allocated 2,000 to 2,500 square feet of space.

If we get the space we then have to have the people. This may involve fundamental decisions on the part of the administration regarding employment practices. So far the hospitals do not seem willing to face the fact that they cannot always get by with cheap labor. Associated with this, of course, is the need for a continuing money supply, and just where this will come from in the medical world is not now clear to me.

Auxilliary facilities, of course, will be necessary, such as animal rooms, clinical lab, pathology, and so on. These will be available in the new hospital complex, though in what quantity is at present not known.

Provision of facilities more appropriate to the physical sciences will remain a major problem. Although it will be desirable to have a good model shop available, I suspect that most of this will have to be done on a more personal basis.

PROFESSOR PETER KATONA

In the past several years we have been involved in the analysis of the carotid sinus reflex, one of the classical control loops regulating blood pressure. Our emphasis has been on the quantitative determination of how changes in blood pressure reflexly influence heart rate. In the course of this work the activity of the pressure receptors and of the cardiac vagal efferent nerves was recorded, and the relationship between these nerve firings and physiologically significant variables (pressure and heart rate) were investigated.

The work was done in Dr. Octo Barnett's cardiovascular laboratory at the Massachusetts General Hospital. Although for a few years the Research Laboratory of Electronics and Dr. Barnett received joint support for this work, liaison between M.I.T. and Massachusetts General Hospital was largely informal. Basically, M.I.T. supplied graduate students, and Massachusetts General Hospital provided the laboratory facilities.

The above activity should be considered as only a step toward the quantitative characterization of the carotid sinus reflex. Future work could progress along two lines. First, it would be interesting to investigate the vasomotor area using microelectrode techniques to determine the physiologic mechanism that is responsible for the observed afferent-to-efferent transformation. Second, by measuring additional relevant variables involved in the regulation of blood pressure (flow, peripheral resistance), a larger portion of the cardiovascular control could be quantitatively characterized. This would aid in understanding the complex interactions involved.

This type of work cannot be continued without increased input from the physiological side. We have lacked the collaboration of a physiologist, whose primary interest is in cardiovascular work and who can devote a considerable portion of his time to the project. The computer facilities (A-D conversion, on-line processing, scope, plotter, and some analogue modules for preprocessing) and laboratory facilities (complete dog lab equipped for nerve recording) have been available at Massachusetts General Hospital, but it would be desirable, though not essential, to have these available at M.I.T.

DR. HOWARD T. HERMANN

I. CURRENT ACTIVITIES: RESEARCH AREAS

A. Signal transfer properties of a specialized interneurone (a single photosensitive unit in the crayfish—small lobster—caudal ganglion). This unit integrates mechanoreceptive inputs from the tail of the animal as well as transducing ambient visible photic energy into an interval-modulated constant-amplitude pulse-train. Closed model formulation of integrative properties is sought. For statistics of intervals we have our own Hewlett Packard 2116A computer with peripherals for A/D input and D/A visual display.

B. Physiology of optic tectum in lower vertebrates (fish, amphibia, and reptile). We are attempting to classify kinds of transformations of data in this visual brain with respect to the information made available to more central decision motor-effector regions. We wish to account for simple predictable classes of motor behavior. We make no effort to handle the data quantitatively.

C. Development of a compact, formal representation of clinical psychiatric phenomena. In effect we are representing what we regard as basic operators in human and animal thinking, with particular reference to clinical psychopathology. We wish to generate a series of clinically useful visual graphic displays (as opposed to the usual linear [auditory] contextually unspecified case presentation). Further, we use the formalism for exposition of strategies in psychotherapy.

Research setting. Our laboratory is relatively isolated from the usual easy cross-fertilization of a compact multidisciplinary research organization (as, for example, in a medical school or the U.C.L.A. Brain Research Institute).

II. PROJECTED PLANS AND ANTICIPATED NEEDS

A. Interneurone signal transfer. Our goals are: (1) analtomical definition of the system; (2) better control of synaptic input; and (3) analysis of membrane fluctuation and ion transfer in context of signal transfer properties. No further implementation of existent computational facilities is needed.

B. Optic tectum. We plan statistical analysis of single-unit responses in order to determine quantitative effects of inputs from other regions of the brain. We shall need to expand our present modest facility with an extra 4K random access memory, dual tape storage (e.g., DECtape), and perhaps high-speed arithmetic if much cross correlation is used. All of this requires an in-house, on-line small computer, or time-sharing with a medium (e.g., PDP9) computer.

C. Psychiatric formalisms. We wish to develop: (1) experimental test situations for study of hypotheses regarding psychopathology; (2) synthetic intelligence simulation embodying features of our theory of human thinking; and (3) a compact graphic storage system for possible computer assistance in planning psychotherapy and epidemiological analysis of clinical material.

In summary, our main anticipated needs are in the realm of synthetic intelligence: simulation and computation facilities, plus the opportunity to interact with scientists more directly involved in such efforts. Overall goal: to relate physiology to behavioral function.

DR. JAMES C. HOUK

PAST AND PRESENT RESEARCH:

1. Mechanisms of mechanoreception, viscoelastic adaptation in muscle receptors, ionic mechanisms.
2. Structural correlates of function in the neuromuscular spindle receptor of mammals.
3. An evaluation of the membrane time constant of spindle receptors from a statistical analysis of discharge patterns.
4. Dynamic characterization of tendon organs in active and inactive muscles.
5. Mathematical model of the stretch reflex in human muscle systems.
6. Measurement of loop gains for force and length feedback control of extensor muscles in the hind limb of the cat.
7. Effects of blocking acetylcholine release on the speed of contraction of fast and slow muscles—trophic determinants of muscle characteristics.
8. Theoretical analysis of fine control in the human thermoregulatory system.
9. Model of the cardiovascular system operating in the steady state.
10. Dynamic characteristics of the vasculature in the hind limb of the dog.

POSSIBLE FUTURE RESEARCH

1. Dynamic characteristics of the stretch reflex in extensor muscles of the cat.
2. The integration of spinal mechanisms for the control of movement.

3. Control of movement by the brain stem and cerebellum.

4. Mechanical properties of single-motor units; recruitment and combination of motor units during muscular control.

5. Effects of use and disuse on the mechanical properties of skeletal muscle.

6. Synthesis of cardiac function from the mechanical properties of heart muscle.

7. Regulation of blood pressure.

FACILITIES:

Ideal facilities for conducting a research program such as I have outlined above would consist of three laboratories, each with access to a small on-line computer, an instrument and electronics room, a room for care of chronic animals, office space for about six people, animal facilities to be shared with other research groups, access to a good machine shop, and the use of large digital and analog computers.

DR. ROBERT J. McLAUGHLIN

1. CURRENT RESEARCH

Present biomedical research by the author concerns dynamic behavior of the cardiovascular and respiratory systems. Several different mathematical models each of mean blood flow (averaged over the pulsatile cycle) and mean ventilation rate (averaged over the respiratory cycle) are being studied analytically and on digital and analog computers, with particular attention to efficient modeling in physiologically meaningful terms and to the particular model ingredients necessary to represent different known dynamic phenomena. Characterization of individual system elements has involved several levels of modeling. For example, ventricular function is being studied by modeling the dynamics of individual phases of the heart cycle in terms of overall ventricle parameters and also in terms of classical cardiac muscle mechanical properties. Appropriate transformations and averages are then utilized to relate models at different levels.

The above research is being conducted in the facilities

of Harvard's division of engineering and applied physics by a research group consisting of the author and four students (three graduate, one postdoctoral). In the past eighteen months six different individuals have been involved and two Ph.D. theses begun in related areas. Computer facilities consist of the division's EAI 680 analog computer and the Harvard Computing Center's IBM 7094 digital machine. Adequate library facilities are vitally important; they are the Harvard Countway Library of Medicine (Boston), libraries of the biology and chemistry departments (Cambridge), and the division's own growing collection in biology and medicine (supported substantially by funds from this project). Experimental data on which to base models has thus far been obtained from published literature, but it is hoped that newly-created ties with the Harvard Medical School may produce other sources.

At least four other faculty members in the division are also doing biomedical research, with the assistance of some of the above and several additional graduate students.

2. FUTURE GOALS

My current interests are in the study of dynamic regulatory processes in the body, mathematical (or control) principles of operation, and the exploitation of this knowledge for clinical use, engineering, design of prostheses or other external systems, and pedagogical purposes. I hope to expand the range of problems both in physiological areas (cardiovascular, respiratory, renal, endocrine, etc.), and in level or depth of study (ranging, say, from membrane and neuron to organ system). Adequate relationships should be established between experimental research activities in physiology and biophysics, clinical medical personnel, persons interested in applying mathematical disciplines, and the engineering world, so that the above research activities will form a bridge from the theoretical to the practical, with useful results of both types and mutual enrichment of all participants.

3. FACILITIES

For such research it is important to have adequate facilities of two rather different kinds: physical and organizational. Physical facilities include machine and electronics shops, digital, analog, or hybrid computers of appropriate size, and secretarial, photographic, drafting, and editorial services. Adequate nearby library resources are important—much time is now lost commuting between Boston and Cambridge for just this. Animal experimental facilities and hospital clinical facilities will also be needed if the above range of theoretical and practical research activities is to be pursued.

It is of at least equal importance to have an organizational structure that will bring into contact people of different backgrounds, in sufficient numbers to make possible meaningful research in this interdisciplinary field. Disciplines such as physiology, neurophysiology, biophysics, biochemistry, applied mathematics, electrical engineering, mechanical engineering, chemical engineering, and computer science may all be involved in bioengineering projects, and the more comprehensive the project, the greater will be the necessity for mutual stimulation from these fields in order to reach the intellectual critical mass for creative, innovative research results. Collaboration can often be arranged through individual initiative within existing structures for cooperation between different departments or institutions, subject to the limitations of physical proximity and financial support. But such collaboration may be tenuous and subject to pressures from the home environments of the collaborators. My experience suggests that it would be very helpful also to have a separate biomedical engineering organizational structure to which individuals would commit some fraction of their time and which would regularly bring all of its members under the same roof. Such a structure, with access to the physical facilities listed above, would bring a distinctly new resource to the individual committed to bioengineering science: a community of other individuals committed to the same enterprise, providing the intellectual climate and resources uniquely favorable to such research.

DOUGLAS R. WAUD

A. CURRENT RESEARCH

I shall describe opportunities for systems analysis in pharmacology rather than just my own interests so as to avoid the personal element. I can classify activities into two groups:

1. Extensions of more familiar physiological studies. For example, once a reasonable model for the cardiovascular control systems is available, one can very easily prescribe drugs to modify the performance of various elements in the system. This, of course, is what is done in the treatment of many cardiovascular disorders. But a systematic, quantitative basis for therapeutic action still needs to be developed.

2. Model building. Here I am thinking of analytical models of theories that have been described qualitatively and require more substantial properties for direct experimental testing. For example, uptake and distribution of drugs (compartmental analysis) obeys a set of equations formally similar to those used in analysis of electrical systems. All the tools developed for this latter activity may easily be carried over to the pharmacological problem, i.e., splitting the system into its component parts, use of transfer functions, and so on. (Note that other approaches are appropriate also.)

B. FUTURE

As you have gathered at our July 1 meeting, I am not sure what the proper approach will be in the future. I am currently interested in seeing if one can train the physician in the appropriate engineering techniques. This still strikes me as the right way around. I am uneasy about training people mechanically in systems analysis and only then looking for a suitable problem.

There are, as I have mentioned, many problems in pharmacology amenable to attack by systems analysis (and other techniques), but I feel that it is the problem that should be central, not an arbitrarily chosen method.

I do not see systems analysis in quite such a central position as do many in the group. For example, in the study of drug distribution, systems analysis is useful but so are ordinary analysis and matrix algebra. I suspect a group oriented toward the systems analytical approach might tend to ignore, for example, the matrix approach.

C. NEEDS

I believe the guiding principle here should be to satisfy the needs of the problem, not the method. Present N.I.H.

policies appear to do this reasonably well inasmuch as support seems to be available for rational projects. I can see that a small library focused on monographs relevant to systems analysis might be handy, but I doubt that it could be placed within easy reach of everyone in the area.

I will add that, as a person in a medical school, I am not as concerned about the absence of facilities for animal research as other members of the group. I believe it would be an error to set up a center for systems analysis in order to get an animal quarters. A physiology department would make more sense and provide the proper outlook as well.

DR. ALFRED D. WEISS

SUMMARY OF CURRENT RESEARCH

1. The project in neurologic correlates of auditory perception uses a system of temporal auditory number judgment in a psychophysical test situation at suprathreshold levels according to a method which has been shown to produce data that can be well characterized by mathematical formulation. There are two aspects to this project. First, these tests are administered to patients with various lesions in the cochlear labyrinth, acoustic nerve, brain stem, and cerebrum. The goal of this aspect of the study is to ascertain the effects of such lesions on the psychophysical response system. The second portion of the study uses a similar but appropriately adjusted psychophysical test utilizing patients that have chronic electrode implants in the temporal lobes. These patients have been implanted because of the diagnosis of temporal lobe epilepsy, and the study under discussion here simply makes use of this patient material. The goal of this portion of the study is to find evoked potential patterns that will, hopefully, correlate with the psychophysical response data that are gathered simultaneously. In this project, cooperation is obtained from the clinical departments of neurology, neurosurgery, otolaryngology, and otoneurology for the supply and clinical assessment of patient material. The department of neurosurgery at the Massachusetts General Hospital supplies the testing facilities for the evoked potential studies, and the psychiatric research laboratory of the Massachusetts

General Hospital provides the computer facilities for data processing.

2. The project in ocular vestibular relationships explores the effects of oscillatory head movements (the head and body being held rigidly) on the ability to maintain visual fixation on a nonmoving point. The effects of different conditions on this system are assessed. Both normal and patient material are tested. Patients are obtained primarily through the otoneurology clinic but in part also from the clinical departments of otolaryngology, neurology, and neurosurgery. The neurophysiology laboratory of the neurology service at the Massachusetts General Hospital provides computer facilities for data processing.

FUTURE RESEARCH PLANS

Future research plans are obviously contingent on the evolution of current projects, the availability of space and funds, and cooperation from other facilities. It is hoped that the first project outlined above will yield a better understanding of how the nervous system processes information, how lesions of sensory and nervous system affect such information flow and processing, and hopefully that it may prove possible to devise methods of recoding information (perhaps by transduction of physical energy prior to sensory stimulation) in such a fashion that it will be possible to bypass or compensate for lesions in the system. The study described in paragraph two on vestibulo-ocular control mechanisms may be expanded to determine vestibular effects on motor systems other than oculomotor, with perhaps an assessment of the interaction between various forms of sensory input with vestibular input on such motor systems.

REQUIREMENTS FOR FUTURE RESEARCH

Aside from the obvious need for space and money, required for any research project, the form of future research depends very much on the kind of ancillary facilities and cooperation that can be obtained from specialists in fields other than my own. The need is to devise and create complex, sophisticated, computer-controlled test systems, create models of functions studied, and apply systems analysis in order to deal with the high-level complexity of the systems involved.

Summary of Activities, Planned Research and Requirements, Field of Physiological Systems Analysis, Man-Vehicle Laboratory, Department of Aeonautics and Astronautics, Massachusetts Institute of Technology, Professors L. R. Young, Y. T. Li, and J. L. Meiry

CURRENT PROGRAMS

1. Mathematical models of the vestibular system, using methods of control theory to relate motions of the head to perceived orientation and nystagmus: experiments on men in rotating and translating devices
2. Mathematical models of the eye tracking system, hybrid stochastic models: experiments on subjects following moving targets
3. Human operator models: multiloop, multi-input models for the pilot, learning and adaptive models, neuromuscular models

FUTURE AREAS OF INTEREST IN PHYSIOLOGICAL SYSTEMS ANALYSIS

1. Control in closed ecological systems
2. Thermal regulation
3. Respiratory control models

CURRENT FACILITIES

Space: 2,500 square feet in Center for Space Research
Hybrid computer ties to various motion devices

REQUIREMENTS (OPTIONAL)

1. Closer ties to electrophysiology laboratory and staff to investigate vestibular connections in cat
2. Animal facilities and operating room for small primates and fish
3. Three-man environmental test chamber and calorimeter including
a Variable atmospheric pressure and gas mixtures
b. Precise control of temperature, humidity, light level
c. Ergometers, physiological monitoring equipment, television, and computer limbs
4. Graphics display terminal with real-time, high-speed access to central computer
5. Moving-base, projected-scene, general purpose vehicle simulator

6. Optics laboratory
7. Standard ophthalmological instrument facility with resident ophthalmologists
8. Machine shop
9. Instrument room (electronic)

Studies of Human Dynamic Space Orientation Using Techniques of Control Theory

ABSTRACT

During the period July 1967 to June 1968, the Man-Vehicle Laboratory pursued a multitude of research topics, all associated with the central problem of understanding and assisting man's orientation in space. Three professors, a full-time research staff member, twelve research assistants partially supported by NsG-577, and five graduate students supported by fellowships or the military participated in associated projects. During this period two ScD. theses and six masters theses were written based on work supported by this grant. The research topics are all concerned with transmission of orientation information to a man, his manual control process thereafter, and the resulting manual output. Our research areas are thus classified according to presentation of information (display research), physiological sensor modeling (vestibular system and eye movements), manual control modeling, and output mechanisms (postural and neuromuscular control). The following areas have been investigated during this past year:

A. Manual control modeling
1. Effects of roll motion cues (Sc.D. thesis)
2. Effects of roll and yaw motion cues (S.M. thesis)
3. Use of variable feel control stick (A.E. thesis)
4. Inverse optimal manual control problems
5. Bayesian learning model for skill acquisition (S.M. thesis)
6. Digital adaptive control (S.M. project)
B. Display research
1. 3-D display development (S.M. project)
2. VTOL integrated display (Sc.D. project)
3. "Anti-vertigo" display (S.M. project)
4. Development of a "head position sensor" (with the Instrumentation Laboratory)

C. Vestibular research
1. Unified model for vestibular function
2. Nonlinearities in rotation sensing (S.M. thesis)
3. Direction preponderance (bias) in semicircular canals
4. Physical modeling of semicircular canals (Sc.D. thesis)
5. Adaptation and habituation (S.M. project)
D. Eye movement modeling
1. Vestibular effects
2. New hybrid model for eye tracking (S.M. thesis)
3. Eye movement in learning to read (S.M. project)
E. Postural and neuromuscular control
1. Research on balance reflex (Sc.D. project)
2. Basic neuromuscular modeling (Sc.D. project—new)
3. Data presentation of muscular activity in skilled action
4. Postural control for extravehicular activity (EVA) propulsion system (new)

Task Group Report on Regionalization of Health Services (Macrosystems)

John F. Rockart
ASSISTANT PROFESSOR OF MANAGEMENT
MASSACHUSETTS INSTITUTE OF TECHNOLOGY, CHAIRMAN

Leona Baumgartner
VISITING PROFESSOR OF SOCIAL MEDICINE
HARVARD MEDICAL SCHOOL

Paul M. Densen
VISITING LECTURER ON BIOSTATISTICS
HARVARD MEDICAL SCHOOL

Martin S. Feldstein
ASSISTANT PROFESSOR OF ECONOMICS
HARVARD UNIVERSITY

Jerome H. Grossman
RESEARCH FELLOW IN MEDICINE
MASSACHUSETTS GENERAL HOSPITAL

James Hartgering
COMMISSIONER OF HEALTH, HOSPITALS, AND WELFARE
CAMBRIDGE CITY HOSPITAL

Osler L. Peterson
VISITING PROFESSOR OF PREVENTIVE MEDICINE
MEMBER OF THE FACULTY OF PUBLIC ADMINISTRATION
HARVARD MEDICAL SCHOOL

Barney Reiffen
LECTURER IN ELECTRICAL ENGINEERING
LINCOLN LABORATORIES
MASSACHUSETTS INSTITUTE OF TECHNOLOGY

Introduction

This memorandum presents the results of the discussions of the macrosystems study group. It is important to note that this report represents a consensus of views and does not necessarily reflect the opinions of any single member.

We define macrosystems as any problem area that involves more than one medical institution—put differently, any problems that exist outside the walls of a single hospital.

Two themes dominated our conversations. First, we are generally concerned that so little work is currently being performed in this area, and we are specifically concerned about the availability of people to perform the work. Our terms of reference did not include the hiring of personnel, so we did not attack the problem. We have no specific commitments from people to undertake the recommended tasks. In general, however, we believe that the attractiveness of the problems selected and of M.I.T. and Harvard as a place to work is such that personnel not now available can be obtained to perform the studies we suggest. In most cases members of this committee or faculty known to us have shown an interest in these problems.

The second theme relates to the site of the work to be performed. We are in complete agreement that the location of the work should be Cambridge wherever possible. To cite the obvious, Cambridge is centrally located; it is a fairly typical city; our group member, Dr. Hartgering, is Commissioner of Health, Hospitals, and Welfare; and it appears that where necessary, good cooperation will be forthcoming from city officials.

We discussed approximately a dozen problems we felt were important in the macrosystems area. They are easily separable into two groups. The first consists of three problems of prime importance, which we suggest should be undertaken by M.I.T. and Harvard. The second group numbers eight problems we believe are of secondary import. A solution for any of this second group will have a minor impact in relation to a solution for a problem of the first group. In many cases, too, work on one of the major problems will automatically include work on one of these second-rank problems.

We recommend that M.I.T. and Harvard undertake programs to:

1. develop a descriptive computer model of the Cambridge medical care system;

2. develop better measures for the rating of effectiveness of changes which are made in the medical care system; and

3. develop a prototype ambulatory care facility.

It should be noted that all of these problems call for the skills of many disciplines. Involved in each should be the efforts of physicians, engineers, scientists, and management personnel.

We believe that our mix of two academic projects and one engineering-oriented demonstration project is a good one. We feel that much research must be done on the descriptive model to obtain a precise understanding of what the medical care system is today. Once the current system is understood, we believe changes to it can be proposed with greater confidence that the changes will be beneficial. Moreover, the model can be utilized to estimate the effects of suggested changes. Experience with modeling has shown this technique to be more effective than the expensive and sometimes devastating "cut and try" methods now used to test new systems.

To estimate the effectiveness of any proposed changes, however, better methods must be developed to measure results. Our measures of the effectiveness of a medical care system today (death/life, number of days hospitalized) are still crude. Intensive effort is needed in this area at this time if changes in the medical care system are to be evaluated with any confidence.

In some contrast with these more academic research efforts, our third recommendation is the development and implementation of a model ambulatory care facility. As we suggest below, ambulatory care is a neglected but increasingly important area of medical care. We believe that the engineering, scientific, medical, and management talents of the M.I.T.-Harvard complex are in a position to make a significant impact on medical care by improving on current efforts in the ambulatory care field and providing a model ambulatory care center to demonstrate what can be done.

The third section presents each of the problems of lesser rank. Finally, the concluding section briefly presents our ideas on the organization necessary to accomplish this work at Harvard–M.I.T.

Three Priority Problems

PROBLEM 1.
DEVELOPMENT OF A DESCRIPTIVE COMPUTER MODEL OF THE CAMBRIDGE CITY MEDICAL CARE SYSTEM

PROBLEM

At this time there is no precise—or even imprecise— model of the medical care system of a major city. The patterns of medical care are seen from isolated viewpoints, and there is no way to assess the impact of suggested changes on the system without actually implementing the change. We believe that the actual pattern of patient care in Cambridge should be modeled—with an attempt made to include the latent demand for as well as current patterns of care.

There is increasing recognition today that health care is a system and that it should be treated as such rather than in the piecemeal basis on which the American health system has been predicated.[1] In addition, there is sufficient understanding of the system to make it generally accepted that changes in one part of a system have sometimes major effects on other parts. Yet changes today are being made in individual parts of the health care system, increasingly disregarding the possible effects on other parts of the system. Furthermore, there are increasing calls for a complete realignment of the system, the need "to develop new patterns for bringing health care to the public."[2] We believe that it is very difficult to predict the *overall* benefit from individual changes that are made or to assess the value of the changes which are made unless the entire existing system is understood.

In other areas, computer models have proved extremely valuable in the understanding of a system and in the forecasting of the effects of changes on the system. The literature is very extensive. To put it simply, models are helpful in two ways: (1) the model provides the designer with extensive insights into the structure of the system itself as the modeling process proceeds; and (2) the model simulates the real world, so suggested changes can be tried and their effects assessed without disturbing the actual situation. Although we believe that it will take extensive effort before a medical care system model can be developed that will be useful for predictive purposes, we believe the insights to be gained from the descriptive step alone will justify the effort.

To date, attempts to model the health care system have been few and limited. Almost all of the efforts have restricted themselves to only a segment of the system; for one example, see.[3] Other attempts have been made on a broad macro-economic scale of econometricians and others.[4,5] At the city level, one descriptive model of Trenton has been developed.[6] Finally, attempts to solve the problem have been made in New York City.[7,8] But New York's complexities make it a tremendously difficult site for the most diligent of modelers. Even in a smaller metropolis, the job of understanding the medical care web is demanding at the least. Medical data sources are available but major problems exist in both the consistency and completeness of data.

These problems notwithstanding, we believe that modeling the health care system in Cambridge is both feasible and of great merit. No case will be made for the fact that Cambridge is in every way an average city. It does, after all, have a very large university component and is a neighbor of one of the world's great medical centers. On the other hand, Cambridge has a population of less than 100,000, a manageable size, a population distribution skewed (like most cities) toward both youth and age, a black ghetto of major proportions, and other attributes that make it representative. Chief among its attributes is that Dr. Hartgering, a member of this study group, is also Commissioner of Health, Hospitals, and Welfare in Cambridge and is deeply interested in seeing this work proceed. Also, data are available in the Cambridge area; sources include the Cambridge hospitals and the relatively advanced record systems of the three major Boston hospitals used by Cambridge residents: Massachusetts General Hospital, Children's Hospital, and the Boston Lying-In Hospital. It is felt there are approximately forty community agencies that would cooperate in this venture. And the Massachusetts Blue

Cross system has an immense amount of Cambridge data.

The modeling process can be carried on at three different levels. The first, and perhaps simplest, of these is the "industrial dynamics" level concerned primarily with the major flows in the system and their feedback effects.[9] This type of model requires the least data gathering but provides an excellent description of the interactions in a system and an overview of its behavior.

At a second level would be a model of a hypothesized Cambridge, using what is known about the population together with the research results of investigators who have defined the behavior of similar segments of other populations (i.e., demand and supply attributes). There are many sources from which these data can be drawn. Blue Cross has extensive data,[10] and there are other studies that can be drawn upon.[11,12] There are studies of post-hospital needs.[13] There is an increasing number of studies of the need for (or the estimated need for) medical care services.[14,15] Finally, there are behavioral studies of selected segments of the population with regard to medical services.[16,17] The list is by no means exhaustive. In general, it is felt that there are enough data available to begin construction of a model, a model that could be helpful at least in determining where interactions do not appear to fit—and therefore, the area in which it is most necessary to gather new data.

At the third level would be a simulation of the medical care system in Cambridge using actual Cambridge data. We have already mentioned possible sources of these data. We have in mind a major simulation effort of the type favored by Amstutz in the pharmaceutical industry consumer modeling process.[18] This model would be by far the most rewarding, it is felt, but will also require the most resources, both human and computer.

COST AND RESOURCES

We feel a feasibility study, of perhaps three months duration, would be necessary to fully establish the feasibility and the ultimate costs of this project. Rough estimates, however, would put the cost of the project, including computer time, at approximately $100,000 for the first-level (industrial dynamics) model, perhaps double that for the second-level model and in the neighborhood of at least \$500,000–\$1,000,000 for the third, and undoubtedly most beneficial, model. We have no particular commitment from faculty to undertake this modeling process at this time, but believe the appropriate faculty and research assistant resources can be found.

We estimate a need for the equivalent of two full-time faculty personnel (divided between the Sloan School and the medical school) as a minimum to direct this work. The equivalent of a half-dozen full-time research assistants and associates will also be necessary over a five-year period to develop the third-level model.

[1] There are a host of references on this subject. For one, see Robert H. Ebert, *Harvard Today*, Spring 1968.

[2] University of Michigan Press Release, Speech of the Surgeon General, November 29, 1967.

[3] Ann D. Peters, and Charles L. Chase, "Patterns of Health Care in Infancy in a Rural Southern County," *American Journal of Public Health*, 57 (March 1967):409–423.

[4] Martin S. Feldstein, "An Aggregate Planning Model of the Health Care Sector," *Medical Care* 5, no. 6, (Nov.–Dec. 1967).

[5] Grover C. Wirick, Jr., "A Multiple Equation Model of Demand for Health Care," *Health Services Research*, 1 (Winter 1966):301–346.

[6] Anne R. Somers, "An American City and its Health Problems," *Medical Care*, 5, no. 3 (May–June 1967).

[7] Nora K. Piore, "Metropolitan Medical Economics," *Scientific American*, 212 (January 1965):19–27.

[8] Paul M. Densen, and Irving Leveson, "Health Accounts: A Proposal Tool for Planning," Unpublished paper, New York City Health Services Administration, Office of Program Planning, Research Evaluation.

[9] Jay W. Forrester, *Industrial Dynamics*, (Cambridge, Mass.: The M.I.T. Press, 1962).

[10] Blue Cross Association, "The Use of Hospitals by Blue Cross Members in 1965," *Blue Cross Reports*, 4 (Oct.–Dec. 1966):1–11.

[11] James C. Ingram and J. D. Colman, "Implications of a Study of the Age Differential in Hospital Costs, *Hospitals*, 41 (March 16, 1967):19–19d, 141.

[12] G. D. Rosenthal, "Factors Affecting the Utilization of Short-Term General Hospitals," *American Journal of Public Health*, 11 (1965):1743.

[13] Merwyn R. Greenlick, Arnold V. Hurtado, and Ernest W. Seward, "The Objective Measurement of the Post-Hospital Needs of a Known Population," *American Journal of Public Health*, 56 (Aug. 1966):1193–1198.

[14] D. Cottwell, Jr., "The Consumption of Medical Care and the Evaluation of Efficiency," *Medical Care*, 4 (Oct.–Dec. 1966):214–236.

[15] Paul J. Feldstein, "Research on the Demand for Health Services," *Milbank Memorial Fund Quarterly*, 44 (July 1966):128–165.

[16] Derek Robinson, "Obstetrical Care and Social Patterns in Metropolitan Boston," *Public Health Reports*, 82 (February 1967):117–126.

[17] Ronald Anderson and Donald C. Reidel, "People and Their Hospital Insurance," Research Series 23 (Chicago: The Center, 1967).

[18] Arnold Amstutz, "The Marketing Executive and Management Information Systems," Working Paper 213–266, Sloan School of Management, M.I.T.

THE PROBLEM

One of the basic difficulties in evaluating changes in medical care is the absence of acceptable criteria for measuring the quantity and quality of care delivered.

The problem is far from simple. There is the subjective question of just what constitutes good medical practice. Even assuming answers to this question, however, presents methods of information collection—medical records preclude the collection of even baseline statistics on the present nature of medical care. Before analytical techniques can be applied, definition of data to be collected and acceptable methods for collection must be developed. However, insurmountable as the problem may seem, it is imperative that techniques for evaluation of care be developed.

This problem is not wholly one of data definition. To codify and standardize data, adequate devices, both from the point of user acceptability and economic feasibility, will have to be developed. Methods of quality control that will monitor on-line the quality of data as they are collected are of great importance.

For example, methods for automated collection of patient medical histories have been developed and tested.[1,2] However, they are economically unfeasible because of the high cost both of terminal devices (CRT or TT) and the central computer system. The development of low-cost terminals for data collection is the key to adequate data collection. This is especially true for the successful enticing of medical personnel into using more structured data-collection formats to register such things as physical findings, diagnoses, and treatments. There is also a need to develop criteria by which such data are to be analyzed, which will deeply influence the nature of the data to be collected.

Some criteria that have been used include the measuring the end results of patient treatment.[3,4] The patient's recovery, residual disability, or death, is determined in relation to the type of treatment or the institutions in which care is given. Studies in upstate New York and in England indicate that there are different case fatality rates following treatment of specific serious diseases depending upon whether care is given in a teaching hospital, another kind of specialized institution, or a community hospital.

However, in other instances, death, disability, or recovery is an inappropriate outcome, since diseases may be self-limited, and postponement of death or prevention of disability is beyond the power of medical treatment. This is particularly true of patients with chronic diseases. In England, where there is regional hospital responsibility, there are clear differences in the efficiency with which chronic disease services cope with the problems of elderly patients, who contribute most to this problem.

It has hitherto been deemed inappropriate to apply some of the more well recognized nonmedical cost/benefit techniques to medicine because of an attitude that medical care—should not be subject to economic considerations. Recently, however, with the ever-spiraling costs of medical care and increasing government participation, it has become clear that a broader viewpoint must be taken in evaluating medical care. This will require economists, sociologists, and management personnel, as well as medical staff, to develop useful criteria. It will also require the status of a prestigious institution to ensure widespread use of any criteria developed. It will require close cooperation with local and national government and the medical community.

FACILITIES AND RESOURCES

This effort's primary requirements will be adequate staff support. The conditions under which the project would operate depend on the affiliations established. Initial support for two faculty-level researchers is indicated.

[1] Warner V. Slack, et al., "A Computer-Based Medical History System," *New England Journal of Medicine*, 274 (January 1966) :193–198.

[2] Jerome H. Grossman, et al., "Medical History Acquisition by Computer," *Hospital Computer Project 1967 Status Report*, (Boston: Massachusetts General Hospital, October 17, 1967).

[3] J. B. Graham and F. P. Palovcek, "Where Should Cancer of the Cervix be Treated: A Preliminary Report," *American Journal of Obstetrical Gynecology*, 87 (October 1, 1963) :405–409.

[4] J. A. Lee, S. L. Morrison, and J. H. Morris, "Fatality From Three Common Surgical Conditions in Teaching and Non-Teaching Hospitals," *Lancet*, 2 (October 1, 1957) :785–790.

A recurring theme in the examination of medical care delivery in recent years has been the call for greater emphasis on ambulatory care. This is reflective not only of the great concern with spiraling costs but also of the organization, efficiency, and efficacy of the care delivered. While the impact of science on medical knowledge has been great,

. . . the provision of care has been little affected by the technological changes. Computers are now a major aid to management in almost every industry, but not in the health care sector. Increasing substitution of capital for labor and advances in communication and transportation have taken place in many service industries, but not in medical care. Yet, it is only exploiting the innovations and technologies of other sectors and by developing new techniques appropriate to its own problems that the health care system can adequately respond to social change and scientific advance.[1]

There have been a few attempts to apply technology in a rational way to medical care. Notable is the Kaiser Permanente Medical Center, especially its multiphasic screening program. These attempts have generally been of limited scope or have been constrained by being add-ons to existing operations. The need exists for a facility geared to innovation and evaluation.

We propose an Ambulatory Health Care Facility (AHCF) that would take full advantage of contemporary technological advances in computers, instrumentation, communications, and system organization. The AHCF would be experimental in nature in that technological innovations would be demonstrated and evaluated in an operating environment. This proposal is related to problem number one, since we believe that the initial step in planning the ambulatory care facility is the understanding of the needs of the community for out-patient care. We also believe that ambulatory facilities should be integrally related with in-patient facilities to provide continuous care. The setting for a new attempt may be in existant institutions or may require the development of an entirely new institution. Among potential existing institutions are the out-patient departments of such hospitals as the Cambridge City Hospital, Beth Israel Hospital, or the Massachusetts General Hospital, or the ambulatory care units planned for Charlestown and the Harvard Prepayment Plan. Each of these presents liabilities, some of size or type of population, others of structure and specificity of function. Therefore, in order to create a more widely applicable and feasible experimental situation, it may be better to develop an entirely new setting.

The concept of a development facility geared to ambulatory care was considered and recommended during the M.I.T. 1967 Summer Study on Engineering and Living Systems. Continued interest within the Harvard and M.I.T. communities has encouraged the evolution of this concept into its present form.

As presently envisioned, the AHCF would include computer-aided history-taking, automated testing, and patient record storage and retrieval. Ultimately it would generalize into tentative diagnoses of selected illnesses and a doctor aid in therapy protocol. The development of the AHCF would proceed in several phases.

1. Initial development of critical components. Collaboration between an engineering center, existing research centers in the Boston area,[2] and several centers of medical excellence (i.e., the teaching hospitals in the Boston area) will guarantee that each component will:
a. be selected on the basis of its clinical relevance in the eventual system;
b. reflect the highest level of medical knowledge;
c. have the preliminary clinical evaluation in a favorable environment, i.e., by the inventor or his close colleagues; and
d. will foster the development of new medical instruments in this manner.

2. Combining the components developed in Phase 1, and other components that may be standard, into the experimental AHCF. This may be viewed as a pilot plant where:
a. evaluation of the components in a less sheltered, more operational, environment is possible;

b. the interrelationship between components will be made evident; and

c. problems introduced by scale (size of operation) can be confronted.

3. In the third phase, the demonstrated capabilities of the AHCF could be projected for replication in other urban areas. This phase aims towards a full prototype of an AHCF. The entire program is thus directed toward growing national needs in the provision of urban health care.

As a facility, the resources of the AHCF need not be dedicated to a single style of health care delivery. Rather, we envision that it should be useful in a variety of situations, such as:

1. In the out-patient department or emergency room of a hospital.

2. For routine work-ups preliminary to or at the time of hospital admission.

3. For routine checkups of asymptomatic populations. This includes annual checkups and multiphasic screening. We make no judgment on the value of these procedures. Rather, we observe that the AHCF can be useful to those medical groups that participate in these procedures.

4. As an aid to physicians in private practice, either in groups or individually. We have in mind special equipment in doctors' offices (consoles and the like) that interface with a remote computer via telephone lines and that can be used for history taking, entry of physical findings, record retrieval, diagnostic and therapy aids, and so on. This capability has the obvious potential of assisting in the postgraduate education of doctors.

The AHCF as outlined above is not restricted to a single physical location. Many consoles may be deployed in doctors' offices and clinics. One or more testing centers may be included, and these would all be interconnected by one or more computers that need not be located in any medical facility.

In Phases 2 and 3, the resources of the AHCF could be devoted to the city of Cambridge, using Cambridge Hospital as a focus. Conditional on availability of resources and interest, the facility can also interface with other existing institutions with a large out-patient population (e.g., Beth Israel Hospital). Similarly, the AHCF could interface with two other ambulatory care units now in the planning stage.

The first is the Harvard Prepayment Plan, sponsored by Harvard Medical School, as a comprehensive prepaid medical care program. The plan proposes to "serve as a framework for systematic investigation of the delivery of medical care and for teaching, studying, and innovating in the provision of health services." [3]

The second is the Bunker Hill Life Services program under the sponsorship of the Massachusetts General Hospital "to provide family-centered health care with comprehensive and continuous services and . . . to utilize technology to the fullest and most realistic extent of the solution of individual and community services." [4]

COST AND RESOURCES

The resources necessary to develop such a facility are significant. They include a large, highly trained, interdisciplinary staff and adequate funding to assure a facility that will be able to attract medical participation.

Starting in September 1968, an intensive, four-month study is planned. The study participants will be individuals from within the Harvard and M.I.T. communities. This study will have as its goal a more specific description of a program leading to an AHCF, including cost and staff implications. We are unable to evaluate full program costs until this study is concluded, which will approximate one to two man-years of effort.

[1] *Report of the National Advisory Commission on Health Manpower* (Washington, D.C., November, 1967).

[2] Such groups as the Laboratory of Computer Science at the Massachusetts General Hospital, and the Systems Group at the Lahey Clinic have been concerned with better methods for the delivery of ambulatory care for a number of years. They serve as an initial repository of information in many of the areas mentioned—i.e., computer-aided history-taking, automated laboratory testing, etc.

[3] *Report to the Dean of Harvard Medical School*, Boston, Massachusetts, August 31, 1967.

[4] *Bunker Hill Life Services Center* (proposal), Boston, Massachusetts, March, 1968.

Problems of the Second Rank

PROBLEM

Despite the ease with which one can compile an extensive bibliography in the area of emergency care, we feel that the problem has not been fully explored nor nearly adequate solutions posed at present.

Cambridge offers an excellent setting in which to work. The city has long had an excellent rescue service supplied by the rescue squad of the city fire department. Training has been provided by the staff of medical schools in the area to update the personnel of the rescue squads in modern methods of resuscitation. As a result, there is a solid basis on which to build further improvements in the system, which currently handles approximately ten cases a day.

Under the direction of Dr. Hartgering, the city has begun an analysis of its emergency care. A study of the patients dead on arrival indicates a substantial number of cardiac cases. It is possible that improved technology could save some of them. The turn-around time of fourteen minutes provides an opportunity for early resuscitation, perhaps by defibrillation.

This is a problem that the Harvard—M.I.T. complex is uniquely able to investigate. The problem is interdisciplinary in that it requires the skills of several branches of engineering, medical, and management personnel. Sample problems include the simple determination of the life or death status of a patient. In addition, if defibrillation is to be considered, the rescue personnel will need to know on a go–no-go basis whether or not the electrical stimulus should be applied.

BUDGET AND PERSONNEL

Current personnel are available to continue the operational aspects of the study, but additional funds will be needed to support technical personnel and to finance equipment development. We are unable to estimate these costs at present.

This problem has been placed in the second rank because of our feeling that it will be considered as part of major Problems 1 and 3.

PROBLEM 5.
EFFECTIVENESS OF COMPUTER-SHARING SYSTEMS

PROBLEM

Hospitals are beginning to share computer systems through telephone lines. The literature reports more than a dozen such efforts. Examples are CHART in New York; EDCO in Wilmington, Delaware; a system sponsored by the state hospital association in Massachusetts; and the multiple hospital system being planned by the Indianapolis Hospital Development Association. The trend toward this interhospital computer sharing has been illustrated and accented by the fact that IBM has developed a software package (Shared Hospital Accounting System) to perform the necessary applications for hospitals involved in a shared system.

These shared systems, when compared to individual hospital computer efforts, would, through economics of scale, be expected to result in lower hardware, software, and system development costs. However, critics of these systems question their responsiveness to the reporting needs of individual managements, the cost of communication equipment, and the ability of individual hospitals to cooperate effectively in a venture of this type.

To the best of our knowledge, although at least one of these systems (CHART) has been in operation for approximately two years and there is an evident trend toward setting up other similar systems, there has been no hard appraisal of the effects—economic or organizational—of shared systems upon the hospitals involved. We believe this should be studied.

COST

The approximate staffing needed would be one faculty member, half-time for a year and two research assistants half-time for a year.

This problem has been placed in the second rank because it can be studied solely by faculty of the school of management.

PROBLEM 6.
MEDICAL DATA BANK FOR LIMITED POPULATION—THE CHILDREN OF CAMBRIDGE

PROBLEM

A child in an urban setting such as Cambridge may see several different physicians or health resources during his first several years. Information available to any of these resources may not be available to others. In the course of his first three years, the child may have been seen by several different physicians. For example, he could have received several of the following, each rendered by a different doctor.

1. Prenatal care
2. Obstetrical care
3. Pediatric care
4. Well-baby clinic care
5. Head start medical care
6. School medical care
7. Private medical care
8. Emergency medical care

In each case, data about the patient will have been entered in a record. Yet in most cases this record will not be available to doctors seeing the patient at a later time. The problem is to evaluate the economics and effect on quality care of providing a readily accessible data bank on the child.

We firmly believe that the major problem here is not the development of the computer techniques to collect and store the data. The primary problem is the determination of whether such a data bank will contribute to the provision of better medical care.

We are aware of much work in the area of computerization of the medical record. Research at Tulane, Roswell Park, New York, Kaiser, and many other places is well recorded. Work is going on at M.I.T.-Harvard's Joint Center for Urban Affairs toward the development of a system. During the past decade, work toward computerization of the medical record has run into many problems, such as coding and the reliability of data. We believe these problems will be overcome eventually. We would advocate a different, and, we believe, more meaningful approach to the problem of the computerization of medical record data—the determination of the need for computerization.

We would propose that a doctor, or nurses and other researchers, working closely with a doctor, evaluate the need for a data bank by following a sample of children through their various medical contacts. They would evaluate whether it would have been helpful for a doctor who perhaps came third in the chain of medical resources to have had available to him the data collected by the first and second physicians. This determination of need would be the first step of the study. Only if the need were found to be present would it be recommended that the more technical, computer-based issues of exact data to be collected and the processing method to be used be studied.

Cambridge's school population is heterogeneous and limited to approximately 1,000 new admissions a year, 85 percent of whom are born in five local hospitals. Children comprise 40 percent of the load of the out-patient department of Cambridge Hospital. Dr. Hartgering has personnel available for assisting in data collection.

The study would have two stages. First, it would be determined whether the presently collected data, if passed on, would have value. Current records, however, leave something to be desired. A second stage, therefore, would be a prospective study of a random selection of children with data input forms designed and supervised.

COST

It is estimated that a feasibility study could be done for about $50,000.

REASONS FOR SECOND RANK

Current efforts of the urban systems group in the field of health information systems make this a possible overlap.

We strongly believe that there is a great need for work in interhospital comparisons. The huge increase in hospital operating costs over the past few years and the expected continuation of this trend underscores the need for this study.

Not estimated.

1. We can discern no interest at M.I.T. or Harvard in this class of problem at present.

2. More importantly, the study of hospital efficiency, particularly when different institutions are compared, has suffered from the lack of information on the diagnosis-mix and other discriminating variables of patients treated. The age of patients, for example, has a profound effect on the number of patients that can be treated per bed per year since the mean stay of patients of age sixty-five or greater is more than twice that of pediatric patients and substantially longer than adults under sixty-five. The proportion of surgical patients will influence hospital costs since preoperative, operative, and postoperative care require more personnel. Even aside from surgical care, the particular diagnosis-mix of patients in a hospital will strongly affect the amount of nursing and other care necessary. In England, Feldstein found that hospital costs were strongly influenced by the case-mix, and this is undoubtedly the case in the United States.

The Massachusetts Blue Cross is at present experimenting with a patient reporting system which will provide data on age, sex, race, discharge diagnosis, length of stay, and other noteworthy characteristics of hospitalized patients. This reporting system currently includes data collection in more than a dozen hospitals, mainly in the Boston area. Its planned extension to cover all hospitals in Massachusetts will provide an opportunity for the first time to obtain a description of hospital inputs, hospital admission rates, case-mixes, and other statistics of interest.

The primary purpose of this reporting system is to provide hospitals with overall utilization rates and utilization rates for each institution. Its extension to all Massachusetts hospitals will require one-and-a-half to two years.

We believe that when the Blue Cross reporting system is operative, a much better base for significant interhospital comparisons will have been built. Perhaps by that time, there will also be more interest in this class of problem generated in the M.I.T.—Harvard complex. We would suggest that the pursuance of this study be postponed until then.

PROBLEM 8.
AN IDEAL SCHOOL HEALTH PROGRAM

PROBLEM

There is distinct dissatisfaction with existing school health programs, especially in cost/benefit terms. Many administrations view current systems as a sink for dollars and personnel. The problems involved are social and political as well as technological and medical. For this reason, an interdisciplinary attack on the development for a better school health system would be desirable.

COSTS

Not estimated.

REASONS FOR SECOND RANK

This problem was discarded early in the discussions because the area is intensely political in nature and clearly not as challenging as the selected problems.

PROBLEM 9.
REVISION OF SYSTEM RULES

PROBLEM

At present there is a well defined set of people (physicians, nurses, and so on) that functions within the health care system. The same can be said about institutions (hospitals of certain types, nursing homes, and the like). The question is whether it is desirable to add new types of personnel or institutions to the system and to revise the functions of the existing participants to provide better health care delivery. (The addition of a less highly or dissimilarly trained "community physician" to take the place of the general practitioner is an example.)

COSTS

Not estimated.

REASONS FOR SECOND RANK

This problem although interesting, is a catch-all for several dozen "role" experimentations that should be performed in the medical setting. We believe the problem to be important, but as a separate problem discounted it since we feel it will be investigated as part of selected Problems 1 and 3.

PROBLEM 10.
IDEAL PATIENT CARE DELIVERY

PROBLEM

The primary medical problem today (in terms of numbers of patients) is not saving life but of caring for patients with chronic problems. In one study only 5 percent of patients came to the doctor with life-endangering problems. Some 30 percent had chronic illnesses and another 65 percent had minor, self-limiting disease. Good nutrition is now turning the emphasis toward care of chronic patients. The question is how to develop the best system to do so. Less fully trained people may be one answer to the need for a cheaper and more responsive medical care system. A second method may be better methods of returning these patients to family care from the acute or chronic disease hospital facilities.

COST

Not estimated.

REASONS FOR SECOND RANK

A solution to major Problem 2 is a necessary preliminary step for judging the effectiveness of efforts in this area. Also it is primarily a medical problem as opposed to an interdisciplinary problem.

PROBLEM

Extended care units in hospitals are not in themselves new. However, recently a type of independent center, typified in the "Children's Inn" at Children's Hospital and the "Medicenters," one of which opened recently in conjunction with Boston University Hospital, has begun to appear. What impact these centers will have, as measured by the criteria of cost, quality of care, and the speed with which patients return to the hospital, is uncertain.

COST

Not estimated.

REASONS FOR SECOND RANK

These centers are still in the earliest stages of development and the few that exist do not constitute adequate volume to call for a major effort at this time.

Organizational Considerations

As a group, we are not unanimous about the best organizational form in which to house the Harvard-M.I.T. efforts. In general, however, we tend to favor a central organization best described as a "loose tent." Each major research activity would be centered in one or a combination of already existing research centers. A central coordinating organization to cover all Harvard-MIT medical care research activities would be created with the following functions:
1. to run seminars for the purposes of education and dissemination of research results;
2. to handle other communication functions;
3. to publish working papers on research results;
4. to provide assistance in obtaining financial support; and
5. to provide policy-making co-ordination.

With regard to the specific projects that we recommend, we can visualize several possible functions for each, as shown in Table 1.

Table 1: Organization of Medical Care Resources

Existing Research Organization	Computer Modelling	Development of Better Result Measures	Ambulatory Center
Harvard Medical Care Research Center (Dr. Densen's Group)	—	X	—
Laboratory of Computer Science (Massachusetts General Hospital)	—	X	X
Urban Systems Group, M.I.T.	X	—	—
Sloan School of Management	X	—	X
Cambridge Department of Health, Hospitals, and Welfare	—	—	X
Other M.I.T. departments	X	—	—
Lincoln Laboratory	—	—	X
Harvard Department of Preventive Medicine	—	X	—

Task Group on Sensory Aids

Robert W. Mann
PROFESSOR OF MECHANICAL ENGINEERING
MASSACHUSETTS INSTITUTE OF TECHNOLOGY, CO-CHAIRMAN

Donald E. Troxel
ASSOCIATE PROFESSOR OF ELECTRICAL ENGINEERING
MASSACHUSETTS INSTITUTE OF TECHNOLOGY, CO-CHAIRMAN

Leslie Clark
DIRECTOR, INTERNATIONAL RESEARCH
AMERICAN FOUNDATION FOR THE BLIND
NEW YORK, N.Y.

Franklin Cooper
PRESIDENT, HASKINS LABORATORIES
NEW YORK, N.Y.

Peter Denes
BELL TELEPHONE LABORATORIES
MURRAY HILL, NEW JERSEY

William Ferrell
ASSISTANT PROFESSOR OF MECHANICAL ENGINEERING
MASSACHUSETTS INSTITUTE OF TECHNOLOGY

Milton Graham
DIRECTOR, AMERICAN FOUNDATION FOR THE BLIND
NEW YORK, N.Y.

Leon Harmon
BELL TELEPHONE LABORATORIES
MURRAY HILL, NEW JERSEY

Kenneth R. Ingham
RESEARCH ASSOCIATE IN ELECTRICAL ENGINEERING
MASSACHUSETTS INSTITUTE OF TECHNOLOGY

Francis F. Lee
ASSOCIATE PROFESSOR OF ELECTRICAL ENGINEERING
MASSACHUSETTS INSTITUTE OF TECHNOLOGY

Patrick W. Nye
WILLIS H. BOOTH COMPUTING CENTER
CALIFORNIA INSTITUTE OF TECHNOLOGY

Vito A. Proscia
CENTER FOR SENSORY AIDS, EVALUATION AND DEVELOPMENT
CAMBRIDGE, MASSACHUSETTS

As stated in the call to the conference, there were three major goals set forth for this committee;
1. to define the term sensory aids in the M.I.T.-Harvard context;
2. to determine what M.I.T.-Harvard can and should do in the area of sensory aids over the course of the next five to ten years; and
3. to determine the recipe for accomplishing these recommendations.

Definition of Sensory Aids

Most of the work at M.I.T. has been concerned exclusively with the blind and almost exclusively with the development of devices and systems to aid the blind. There have been three distinct groups at M.I.T. concerned with sensory aids: the Research Laboratory for Electronics (RLE), the mechanical engineering department, and the Center for Sensory Aids Evaluation and Development (CSAED). Summaries of their respective research objectives are listed in Appendixes 1A, 1B, and 1C. Obviously, sensory aids could easily entail aids for the deaf as well as the blind, and there are many interesting research opportunities concerned with the problems of the deaf. While this is a reasonable area for expansion of interest in sensory aids, it does not appear that there is a great desire on the part of present M.I.T. personnel to initiate such research.

Since sensory aids transfer the environmental sensing burden from one modality to another, study of all potential human sensory alternatives is unavoidable. Furthermore, demographic data indicate that single sensory deprivation is less prevalent than cases of multiple impairment. Thus, future effort in sensory aids at M.I.T. may become less specialized with respect to the blind.

What to Do and How

The following possibilities are listed in ascending order of the funding required. This order also reflects perhaps the degree of interest of the M.I.T. personnel who might be involved.
1. The very least that could be done is to maintain the status quo. Presumably, this requires zero additional

funds. That is, we now have viable research groups in the electrical and mechanical engineering departments that are nurtured by interested faculty and will continue to produce new ideas and approaches to the problems of sensory aids for the blind. There also exists the M.I.T. Center for Sensory Aids Evaluation and Development. While this center is minimally funded, it does serve as an important contact with the blind community, and can provide (for fairly small projects) some of the necessary development and evaluation of sensory aids prototypes.

2. The availability of possibly as little as $100,000 or less per year could provide a significant boost to the productivity of the three existing M.I.T. groups. Perhaps the place where money is most urgently needed is the Center for Sensory Aids Evaluation and Development. Additional funds on this order could enable the actual prototype development and evaluation of projects concerning, for example, braille distribution and compressed speech.

3. A considerably more ambitious undertaking that might be housed within a new organization would involve the creation of a research and development group dedicated to solving the problems of blind mobility. Such an undertaking would necessarily require a two-to three-year instrumentation development effort and the acquisition of a large computer (e.g., a PDP-10) to realize an adequate simulation facility (See Appendix 2). A rough estimate of its cost would be $600,000 for the first year and $400,000 per year for each of the succeeding four years. It would require a full-time staff of an electrical engineer, a mechanical engineer, a psychologist, two programmers, and supporting personnel. Of course, interested faculty and graduate students would be involved in the design of such a simulation facility and would make use of the system to conduct experiments on mobility, man-machine systems, and sensory modality transfer. A central feature of this research and development operation would be the involvement of the blind community in evaluation and acceptance studies by the permanent staff. It is in these directions that future expansions of the sensory aids group would be most likely. The Research Laboratory, of Electronics, the mechanical engineering department, and the Center

for Sensory Aids Evaluation and Development all see the mobility simulation as a project of mutual interest in which they are prepared to collaborate.

Two recent reports outline the problems of providing sensory aids for the blind and deaf respectively and indicate the present status and future requirements of research in these areas. The National Research Council report, (Appendix 3) among its recommendations, proposes:

"Several research centers combining the mutually beneficial resources of university and industrial organizations capable of making contributions to fundamental and applied research and development (in sensory aids)."

The M.I.T. sensory aids program might very well evolve into such a center, perhaps as part of a bioengineering center.

In order to support larger scale investigations and carry through engineering development and evaluation, such a center presupposes a higher ratio of professional staff to faculty-graduate student participation than is common in academically-based projects. Appendix 3 includes a discussion of these problems in the context of sensory aids.

Appendix IA:

RESEARCH OBJECTIVES AND SUMMARY OF RESEARCH OF THE COGNITIVE INFORMATION PROCESSING GROUP OF THE RESEARCH LABORATORY OF ELECTORNICS, M.I.T.

The primary research interest of this group is in the real-time acquisition and processing of visual information for display to the visual and nonvisual senses and in the psychology of human utilization of such information for both communication and control. The motivation is an interest in human capabilities for information processing and in human information requirements. Applications include sensory aids systems for the blind and the blind-deaf, picture-transmission systems, and special information-display systems for enhancement of human performance under conditions of stress.

Major projects now in progress include studies on reading machines, picture processing, pattern recognition, and automatic processing of visual data of significance in studies of biology and medicine. Following is a description of the research areas connected with sensory aids for the blind.

READING MACHINE STUDIES

Research during the past few years in the cognitive information processing group of the Research Laboratory of Electronics has led to the construction and operation of an experimental reading system for the blind. In its present configuration, the system consists of a document-handling carriage, a flying-spot opaque scanner, a digital scanner control unit, and a general-purpose medium-sized computer (PDP-1). Focusing, black-and-white threshold setting, and document loading are manually controlled by a sighted operator. The scanner control unit, operating under control of the computer program, reports coordinate letter contour and other statistical information of the view in the scanner field. This information is used for the generation of signatures that are searched in a signature table for identification of the letters. The signature table is built up through training sessions. Identified letters are spelled out one at a time through digitized speech samples. The present output rate of the spelled speech is sixty to eighty words per minute. Experience has indicated an identification error rate of approximately 0.3 percent with a type font that the machine has been trained on.

Another objective for future research is to evaluate the reading machine under conditions of actual use by blind subjects. For this an improved input system that allows the use of books in their normal form is needed.

CHARACTER RECOGNITION

A new character recognition algorithm has been devised and tested. The preliminary results of this algorithm, which involved the determination of extrema along the x, y, $x + y$, and $x - y$ axes, are quite encouraging, and a more rigorous evaluation is in progress.

The character-recognition algorithm used in the reading machine system has been tested on printing containing touching letters. A recursive procedure was employed with good success. The problem of broken letters is yet to be investigated.

OPAQUE SCANNERS

A new opaque scanner with a wider field of view and an improved document handler is in the final phases of construction. A scheme for reading specified portions of a vidicon television camera into computer memory is in the design phase. A longer term goal is the construction of a hand-held probe, utilizing fiber optics to couple the print image to the vidicon camera.

TACTILE DISPLAYS

A 6×8 matrix of solenoid-powered poke probes has been interfaced to the PDP-1 computer. Under construction is an electrotactile matrix display that will be used to study both static and dynamic tactile perception.

TRANSFORMED SPEECH

Experiments are being planned to determine whether subjects are able to learn to recognize transformed speech. The transformation to be considered in the first set of experiments consists of inverting the spectrum of speech utterances, i.e., $T(f) = 1/f$, and playing back the inverted speech to the subjects.

PHONETIC TRANSLATION OF ENGLISH TEXT AND ARTIFICIAL-SPEECH

Artificial-speech generation from input consisting of English sentences in normal spelling was successfully accomplished in March 1967. The implementation then bypassed the syntactic analysis and made use of only lexical stresses and punctuation marks for suprasegmental control. Since then, work has been concentrated in two areas. The first is the search of a minimal syntactic analysis consistent with the reading-machine objective. The second is the improvement of speech quality within the limitations of our speech synthesizer.

REAL-TIME, DATA-PROCESSING FACILITIES

A PDP-9 computer has been ordered, which will serve the real-time data-processing needs of our entire group. All activities associated with the reading-machine project will be transferred to use in the new facility.

Also, the problem of machine-aided speech recognition through operations on speech spectrograph data, will be investigated. A logical unit to perform Fourier transforms at high speed is under design consideration, to be an important element of the real-time, data-processing facilities.

Appendix 1B:
A READING MACHINE FOR THE BLIND

D. E. TROXEL
RESEARCH LABORATORY OF ELECTRONICS
MASSACHUSETTS INSTITUTE OF TECHNOLOGY

F. F. LEE
RESEARCH LABORATORY OF ELECTRONICS
MASSACHUSETTS INSTITUTE OF TECHNOLOGY

S. J. MASON
RESEARCH LABORATORY OF ELECTRONICS
MASSACHUSETTS INSTITUTE OF TECHNOLOGY

At present, the blind use two means of reading that do not require the assistance of a sighted person—Braille and prerecorded spoken material. The long time lag, inherent in these partial solutions, between the desire to read a particular passage and the availability of the prepared material is a distinct disadvantage. Printed matter such as newspapers and periodicals cannot be effectively read by these methods. The reading machine [2] under development at M.I.T. would allow the blind reader immediate access to the bulk of existing printed matter.

METHOD

Our approach is based on the recognition of individual characters by the machine and their immediate presentation to the blind reader in the form of spelled speech. The equipment for performing these tasks includes a document-handler, a flying spot opaque scanner, a special-purpose digital system termed scanner controller, a data link to a medium-sized general-purpose digital computer, along with audio display for a blind reader and suitable visual displays for a sighted operator.

The light source for the opaque scanner is an oscilloscope whose deflection voltages are supplied by the scanner controller. This dot of light is imaged on the paper by a single lens, and the diffuse reflected light is collected by two photomultiplier tubes. The absence of signal from the photomultiplier tubes indicates that the particular spot on the page as specified by the oscilloscope deflection voltages is black. The present system requires adjustment of focus, threshold, and initial paper position by a sighted operator. When these adjustments are satisfactory, the blind person initiates the reading process. The computer program delivers a succession of commands to the scanner controller and processes the returned data to determine the base and mid lines of a line of text (e.g., the top and bottom of a small e). Next, the first letter of text is acquired, its contour is traced, and a list of edge point coordinates is transmitted to the computer. A characteristic number or signature is then computed for this contour by determining both the vertical extent of the contour with respect to the base and mid lines and the horizontal and vertical extrema, along with the quadrants in which each occurs. The last step in the recognition process involves a search of a code table, which is a summary of the previous training of the machine.

APPLICATIONS

The reading machine has been fully trained on one Roman type font and recognizes lower and upper case letters, numbers and punctuation marks. The only accuracy run, thus far, yielded three errors in approximately 950 successive characters of text. The spelled speech which forms the audio output has been preprocessed so that the maximum output rate is 120 words per minute. As the character-recognition process is alternated with the output of the recognized letters, the average speed of the machine is approximately 80 words per minute, which is comparable with that of Braille. Collateral tests of the spelled speech employed have indicated that blind subjects can learn to understand presentations at the 120 word per minute rate with approximately 10–20 hours practice.

The immediate application of the reading machine is to serve as a research vehicle for the development and refinement of (a) character recognition algorithms, (b) methods to enable the blind reader to adjust various necessary controls that cannot be economically automated, and (c) alternative methods of output of the text material such as synthesized speech or Braille.

While of course, this procedure does not restore sight to the blind, it does offer a prosthesis for reading problems. The availability of reading machines such as this, even if limited to library use, would enable the blind to have access to printed matter essentially equivalent to that available to the sighted. The system is complex, but we expect that advances in the state of the art of digital systems will allow a considerably more economical implementation of a reading machine in the future. Training is in progress on several other fonts, including newsprint and typewritten material.

[1] Reprinted from *Digest of the 7th International Conference on Medical and Biological Engineering*, Session 26, "Aids for the Handicapped" (Stockholm, 1967).

Appendix 2: Research Objectives of Mechanical Engineering Department Sensory Aids Group

Studies directed toward enhancing information acquisition of the blind. Research on audiotactile and kinesthetic stimuli and their effectiveness in information transmittal.

Use of new techniques to record—simultaneously—lip position and shape, breath pressure, larynx and nasal frequencies, and so on, to help the deaf-blind. This procedure permits the analysis of speech aspects not observable using the usual frequency techniques.

BLIND MOBILITY DEVICE EVALUATION AND SIMULATION

Research and development of subject tracking and data acquisition and processing and display schemes, whereby the effectiveness of blind mobility aids and the competence of blind mobility trainees can be evaluated. The system is also intended for the simulation of potentially useful mobility devices. It provides computer-generated displays through which the simulated device describes the obstacle environment to the man.

BRAILLE TRANSLATION AND COPY PREPARATION

Evaluation of a remote-access, English-to-braille translation system. Using computer programs for the translation as well as machines which emboss braille at electric typewriter speeds, the system incorporates a centralized computer and a communication network of ordinary telephone lines.

BRAILLE PRINTING DEVICES

Design and development of a high-speed electric braille typewriter to be operated by computer output, punched paper tape, keyboard, or an attachment to an ordinary office typewriter.

TAPE-TO-BRAILLE MECHANICAL TRANSDUCERS

Design and development of tape-to-braille mechanical transducers utilizing perforated and/or magnetic tape as an input to set a continuous line of braille characters on a moving belt.

Appendix 3A:
SCOPE OF ACTIVITIES OF THE M.I.T. SENSORY AIDS EVALUATION AND DEVELOPMENT CENTER

A facility to evaluate and further develop communication, mobility, vocational, and other aids for the blind and deaf-blind. The center keeps abreast of national and international research and development of preprototype processes and devices. Promising approaches are evaluated through psychophysical evaluation programs using blind and deaf-blind subjects from the Boston area. Concurrent development and improvements suggested by the testing are carried out at the center, including production engineering where appropriate. Devices and processes that prove useful to the blind and deaf-blind are brought to the attention of industry, government, and agencies for the blind.

In addition to the director, the center staff includes a psychological and engineering staff, plus supporting administrative and technical aides. A steering committee to formulate policy, define projects, and approve recommendations is comprised of faculty and research staff in engineering, science, psychology, and social work. A national advisory committee of experts in the pertinent fields meets periodically with the center staff and steering committee.

Appendix 3B:
A COMPREHENSIVE, COMPUTER-BASED, BRAILLE TRANSLATING SYSTEM

R. W. MANN
DEPARTMENT OF ENGINEERING
MASSACHUSETTS INSTITUTE OF TECHNOLOGY

The supply of Braille, essential to the blind's acquisition of reading skills and their assimulation of concise, symbolic, format organized (tabular, etc.) and private information, has been extremely limited in scope and currentness. The unrelenting expansion of the blind population due to population growth and longevity multiplies the demand for Braille. The information "explosion" proliferates the knowledge to which the blind need access. Contemporary rehabilitation policies recognize that the blind must function in the world of the sighted, opening up new vocational and recreational opportunities. These conditions make mandatory the facilitation of information flow to the blind through the exploitation of data processing techniques developed for other fields.

METHOD

Since 1959, a faculty and student group in Mechanical Engineering at the Massachusetts Institute of Technology [2] and since 1964 the Center for Sensory Aids Evaluation and Development also at M.I.T., both sponsored by the Vocational Rehabilitation Administration of the U.S. Department of Health, Education and Welfare, have been developing a system which will expand the volume and variety of Braille encoded information while reducing the processing time. A central computer with a translation from English to Grade II (contracted) Braille program (BRAILL) and an input accommodation and formal organization program (DOTSYS) accepts any of several inputs and drives any of several paper embossing outputs depending upon the kind of information to be processed and the rapidity with which results are desired.

The information the blind desire in Braille can be characterized as: 1) widely circulated, lengthy, ink-print publications (books, texts, popular periodicals, etc.); 2) very limited circulation, lengthy, ink-print publications (professional journals, reports, etc.); 3) single or few copy, short unpublished material (notes and correspondence, student homework and examinations, etc.).

For categories 1 and 2, commercial, ink-print publication produces encoded information used to automatically set type. Type-compositor's tape readers can automatically decipher and provide computer input for any ink-print material for which the tape record is still available, a process far more economical and practical than the use of still very limited and costly character recognition machines. Teletypesetter tape used in the linotype process is processed by standard tape readers. Monotype tape requires a new reader now virtually operational. For category 3, information input in ordinary English is by typewriter keyboard generating electrically coded signals.

256

At the output, embossing of category 1 information, when volume production is desired, will continue to be done by press embossing methods. For category 2 information, when one or several copies will suffice, but speed of delivery is important, the conversion of a standard computer chain-printer produces intelligible-to-perfect embossed Braille depending upon the refinement of the conversion unit. Such conversion does not interfere with the normal alphanumeric use of the printer. For category 3 (and perhaps category 2) information, an electric-typewriter-speed-and-size Braille Embosser is located with the blind person, remote from the central computer, using standard telephone connections. An alternative, portable, less costly Braille-Belt display accepts computer-punched paper tape and presents Braille continuously. An input keyboard permits preparation and proofreading of punched paper tape for later rereading or mailing to a similarly equipped person.

APPLICATIONS

Teletypesetter tape into embossed Grade II Braille has been demonstrated to the satisfaction of a critical audience of Braille users. Monotype tape conversion will be in operation this fall (1967).

The typewriter-like Braille Embossers have been in use for over a year, one by a blind computer expert who receives his print-out in Braille. Another is in use in a school for the blind. This fall several units in public and residential schools in the Boston Metropolitan area will service the Braille translation needs of students and teachers, connected by telephone lines to the M.I.T. computer. In the interactive, real-time multiple-access mode, keyboard operation at the school produces virtually instantaneous embossed Braille at the school. In the batch processing mode, small lots of monotype tape input at M.I.T. produces desired text material in Braille at the school. The Brailler may be capable of direct production of zinc plates for press embossing.

The Braille-Belt display, still under development, has had limited use in kinesthetic studies of Braille reading and has been well received. They may be particularly useful to the deaf-blind who could thus receive current information daily.

DISCUSSION

The technical feasibility of most aspects of the overall system has been demonstrated. Wide-scale deployment depends upon market demand and the economics of device production and computer service.[3]

[1] Reprinted from *Digest of the 7th International Conference on Medical and Biological Engineering*, Session 126, "Aids for the Handicapped" (Stockholm, 1967).

[2] R. W. Mann (1962). "Enhancing the Availability of Braille," *Int. Cong. Tech. and Blind.*, A.F.B., N.Y.

[3] L. H. Goldish (1967). "Braille in the U.S., Its Production, Distribution and Use." *Research Bulletin*, A.F.B., N.Y.

Appendix 4:
THE EVALUATION AND SIMULATION OF MOBILITY AIDS FOR THE BLIND [1]

ROBERT W. MANN
MASSACHUSETTS INSTITUTE OF TECHNOLOGY

INTRODUCTION

Earlier work on blind mobility research in the Mechanical Engineering Department at Massachusetts Institute of Technology (M.I.T.), under the Vocational Rehabilitation Administration, Department of Health, Education, and Welfare sponsorship, has focused on the information transmission characteristics of the long cane and the study of obstacle course negotiation by blind travelers (6). This experience and our cognizance of the work of other investigators concerned with blind mobility devices, such as the Haverford/Bionic infrared probe (2) and the Kay/Ultra (3) and Russel ultrasound probes (4) convince us that the most crucial, least understood and, therefore, most challenging aspect of the overall blind-mobility-assist problem is that of the display and assimilation by the user of the information acquired by the instrument.

SEARCH AND DETECTION

Progress to date by other investigators has already adequately demonstrated that the technical aspects of search and obstacle detection can be accomplished through use of optical or sonar techniques. While refinements beyond present capabilities are essential, the means by which to realize such improvements can be mustered when the utility of the devices to the blind can be demonstrated.

Similarly, problems of bulk, weight, complexity, and reliability of the power supply, signal gathering, receiving, discriminating, amplifying, and so on, elements of present instruments are not very satisfactory, and quite remarkable improvements are possible when the concomitant usefulness can be justified. Striking progress in solid state devices, microelectronics, battery research, etc., undertaken for reasons quite foreign to the problems of blind mobility are, and will be directly applicable.

DISPLAY

Thus the central and pervading problem is that of the means of display to the traveler of his environment through sensory modalities ill-equipped relative to the speed, comprehensiveness, and spatial resolution of the human eye. Part of the display problem (and difficult of segregation from the art of beholding) is the discrimination in the field of view of objects of especial and timely interest for the blind man, i.e., the obstacles he must avoid or comply with.

It is our considered opinion that the purely technical aspects of mobility assists—search, size, reliability, and so forth, but excluding display—are realizable, but not without considerable development time and expenditure of resources for each and every device. The really unresolved questions are the modes and forms of display and the human's reaction to, effective assimilation of, and response to the display. In recognition of this gap, we have directed our sensory measurements research to the study of a system by means of which we hope to be able to simulate the essential attributes of the environment-device-man mobility assist situation without our, or others, undertaking the time-consuming and expensive detailed design development, and test of specific devices.

MOBILITY AID EVALUATION

A more immediate, but happily closely related problem is that of systematical, rational, and fair evaluation of mobility aids as they become available. The measure of the utility of an aid goes quite beyond a subjective opinion on the part of a user. We need to know how the aid helps the user respond to a great variety of travel situations, how a spectrum of blind travelers of different competences respond to the aid, and how training with the aid enhances its usefulness.

COMPUTER ORGANIZATION OF MOBILITY PERFORMANCE

The data processing capability of a modern high speed computer can, in principle, be organized to maintain a space-coordinate/time record of a human as he negotiates obstacles. The obstacles themselves might not exist

TASK GROUP REPORT ON SENSORY AIDS

physically, but only in the computer's memory of the environment coordinate space. On the basis of input information on the man's position, the computer could be programmed to calculate the man's relationship to the "obstacle." On the basis of criteria defining the characteristics of a simulated detection device the computer could generate a signal which represented the device's interception of the obstacle. This signal could, in turn, be presented to the man in some physical fashion, transmitted from the computer by means of cable or radio to a portable display.

Thus, the "device," except for the display, is completely simulated. "Device" search characteristics such as range, field of view, scanning routine, resolution, and the like, are determined within the computer by suitable programming, permitting these characteristics to be easily and rapidly altered.

With such a computer centered scheme, systematic tests varying significant parameters of different guidance device concepts could be rapidly, efficiently, and objectively conducted without the expensive, time consuming detailed design, development, and fabrication of each variation of each class of device.

As a by-product of the simulation role, the computer provides an invaluable bookkeeping function as an indefatigable, errorless, unprejudiced observer and recorder of the man's effectiveness in coping with the obstacle using this particular setting of this particular class of mobility device. Thus the difficult, time consuming, opinionated, and often ambiguous task of man-device evaluation is regularized and organized.

The combination of the device simulation role and the evaluation recording capability of the computer system suggests the prospects of extraordinary advances in the delineation of design goals and specifications and the comparison and ranking of the utility of alternative mobility devices. Beyond these direct applications, such a system would constitute a powerful research instrument for the study of mobility itself.

SUBJECT TRACKING SCHEMES

In view of the evaluation/bookkeeping promise of this approach, and its obvious extension to training and rehabilitation programs built around device utilization,[2] we have concentrated thus far on the physical means by which the coordinate position of a subject could be tracked, and the concomitant problem of computer manipulation of the input so as to provide a record of the subject's path through the obstacle space.

With a view toward the realization of a tracking method and, ultimately, environment/device simulation, compatible with both the evaluation of current (or soon to be realized) devices, we established design goals of:

1. simultaneous tracking of several points on the subject (i.e., head, "mobility device," right foot, etc.) ;

2. object field large enough to permit realistic situations;

3. feasibility and availability of tracker combined with compatibility with computer input and calculation routine;

4. satisfactory resolution of the geometric and dynamic relationships between man and obstacle; and

5. minimum impediment to the subject.

The most promising scheme considered thus far by the Mechanical Engineering Sensory Aids Group at M.I.T. uses a military surplus stabilized platform on which a star tracker is mounted. The star tracker detects an infrared or visible light target attached to points of interest on the subject and provides error signals to the stablized platform devices, which, in turn, keep the tracker aligned on the targets on the subject. Resolvers on the platform axes feed angular information into the computer where simple trigonometric calculations generate the x, y, and z coordinates of the path of the target point of interest.

Discrimination among several targets on the man and device—hand, head, etc.—could be accomplished by using different spectral emissions and appropriate filtering, or by means of polarization techniques.

With two such trackers on poles of reasonable height, the path of a subject could be observed over a football field area. A third tracker would provide a redundancy check and ensure against tracking loss due to temporary obscuration of the target.

After a study of system requirements by Mr. David R. Stoutemyer, a research assistant conducting the investigation and consultation with faculty and professional colleagues active in inertial and celestial navigation, a military surplus platform has been obtained and experiments with it are under way (7). The equipment presently under development could be used both as the input for a research investigation of man-device display and interaction, and could also be used for the direct evaluation of extant sensory mobility devices.

My colleagues at M.I.T. in Professor Samuel J. Mason's group in the Research Laboratory of Electronics have taken a somewhat different approach to the tracking problem. Mr. Emanuel Landsman is studying the use of ultrasonic signals with a sound generator sited on the subject and three microphones located in the test space. Calculations of the phase shift at the receivers between the arrival of the pulses from the subject provides trigonometric data on subject location.

COMPUTER PROCESSING

The computer resolution of tracker input information into the space/time location of the subject is a straightforward problem, as is the generation within the computer of spatial parameters representative of the search pattern of the simulated detection device. The task of instructing the computer to recognize and define the interaction between the "volume" simulating an obstacle and the "volume" swept by the device detector is not trivial, especially when one faces up to problems of resolution, real-time calculation, and limited computer memory capacity. The work of Dr. Larry G. Roberts of Lincoln Laboratory, M.I.T., in programming a computer to display the merging of solid objects is certainly relevant. Mr. R. M. Baecker in electrical engineering has also explored this problem (1).

TACTILE AND AUDIO DISPLAY

The computer processing of tracking and detection will permit great freedom in the choice and study of alternative displays and combinations of displays to the human. This part of the overall system must of course be physical since it must interact with the man. But since the signals driving the display will be computer originated it will be easy to preprocess, integrate, or modulate the signal in a wide variety of ways while still in the computer itself. Then the output can be transmitted to the display via cable or telemetry link. Since the display itself will be free of the interconnection and geometry restrictions imposed on a real detection device, it can tend toward a universal capability rather than being warmly specific. One can visualize spatially distributed tactile transducers operable at different frequencies, pulse rates, amplitudes, and so on, combined perhaps with monaural and binaural audio displays, again with variable frequency, amplitude, phasing, and the like, and coding capability.

In the final analysis, this is the heart of the mobility problem. How does one impedance match a remaining sensory modality of a human being, or some combination of modalities, with a stimulation so as to provide the most satisfactory characterization of his environment to a blind man?

THE MAN-MACHINE SYSTEM

Armed with his display and confronting his imaginary obstacles, the man completes the loop—from the man-held simulated detection device, to computer, to display, and then through the man's reaction to his presumed obstacles back to the computer via the tracker.

The overall simulation scheme presents an enormous increase in our ability to understand and master the problems of blind mobility. But it must also be noted that the realization of the comprehensive plan represents a very large effort and the deployment of very substantial resources. The work currently under way must be recognized as fragmentary and explorative, a search to define feasibility and the optimum methods for handling components of the over-all system. In light of the necessarily progressive nature of the study, it is especially important, I believe, that the design be carried forward in such a way that elements of the system have utility of and by themselves, especially as described earlier in the context of evaluation of real mobility aids already with us, some of which were described and demonstrated at the Rotterdam Mobility Research Conference.

Footnotes

---

[1] This paper was originally presented at the Rotterdam Mobility Research Conference, published in *Research Bulletin*, No. 11 (October 1965), American Foundation for the Blind, New York City.

² Note the obvious relationship between this capability and the mobility device program of the center for sensory aids evaluation and development described elsewhere (5).

References

1. Ronald M. Baecker, "Computer Simulation of Mobility Aids—A Feasibility Study." Unpublished Master's thesis, Department of Electrical Engineering, Massachusetts Institute of Technology, Cambridge, Massachusetts, 1964.

2. Bruce H. Deatherage, "The Evaluation of the Haverford-Bionic Instruments Obstacle Detector," L. L. Clark, ed., *Proceedings of the Rotterdam Mobility Research Conference* (New York: American Foundation for the Blind, 1965), pp. 201–233.

3. Leslie Kay, "Ultrasonic Mobility Aids for the Blind," in L. L. Clark, ed., *Proceedings of the Rotterdam Mobility Research Conference* (New York: American Foundation for the Blind, 1965), pp. 9–16.

4. L. Russell, "Travel Path Sounder," L. L. Clark, ed., *Proceedings of the Rotterdam Mobility Research Conference* (New York: American Foundation for the Blind, 1965), pp. 73–78.

5. Robert W. Mann, "The Establishment of a Center for Sensory Aids Evaluation and Development," L. L. Clark, ed., *Proceedings of the Rotterdam Mobility Research Conference* (New York: American Foundation for the Blind, 1965), pp. 173–190.

6. T. B. Sheriden, "Techniques of Information Generation: The Cane," in L. L. Clark, ed., *Proceedings of the International Congress on Technology and Blindness*, Vol 1 (New York: American Foundation for the Blind, 1963), pp. 13–34.

7. David R. Stoutemyer, "Systems Study and Design of a Blind Mobility Aid Simulator." Master's thesis, Department of Mechanical Engineering, Massachusetts Institute of Technology, Cambridge, Massachusetts, 1965.

Appendix 5:
EXCERPTS FROM "SENSORY AIDS FOR THE BLIND," REPORT AND RECOM-
MENDATIONS, SUBCOMMITTEE ON SENSORY AIDS, COMMITTEE ON PROS-
THETICS RESEARCH AND DEVELOPMENT, NATIONAL RESEARCH COUNCIL,
MAY 1967 PUBLICATION 1691, NATIONAL ACADEMY OF SCIENCE

FOREWORD

The purpose of this report is to outline the current state-
of-the-art of sensory aids for the blind, to cite inadequacies in past efforts and funding to provide technological
supplements, and to document areas of research, development, evaluation, and deployment which are required
to meet more satisfactorily the requirements of the blind.
Reflecting on past experience we formulate plans for a
greater effort to provide rehabilitation for the blind at
the individual, vocational, industrial, and national levels. We are convinced that such an effort is warranted on
a humanitarian basis, but we do not overlook the ultimate compensation of program costs through the increased earning power of the rehabilitated blind and
visually impaired.

Specific recommendations define an effective, sus-
tained, integrated, long-range program:

1. The scientific, technological, rehabilitation and
economic resources of the nation must be mobilized to
provide an effective program to meet the needs of the
blind. Such a program should embrace research, development, and evaluation of blind aids, and eventual deployment and training in their use.

2. Three major thrusts of basic research are required:

a. assessment of information requirements of the blind;
b. assessment of human perceptual and sensory capabilities; and
c. technological studies on the acquisition, processing,
and display of information.

3. The systematic evaluation of sensory aids to determine utility, to guide research, to feed back information
for redesign, and to establish valid training procedures
is mandatory and must be carried out in close liaison
with research efforts.

4. The developmental facilities and costs associated
with the production of small, experimental lots of prom-
ising-devices must be recognized and provided for, as

must the ultimate production engineering, operational, and maintenance aspects of deployed devices and sytems. Concurrent demographic and economic studies must explore the cost benefit prospects of prospective devices and systems to plan adequately for deployment costs and organization.

Assessing the present state-of-the-art we recommend program priorities:

1. Emphasis should be placed on the reading problem because of the present promise of early significant results that will require substantial developmental efforts.

2. A concerted attack on the mobility problem should proceed concurrently with that on the reading problem, but owing to our ignorance of human mobility (compared to reading) and the need for experience with man-device interaction, research, and small-scale evaluation should be emphasized.

3. A strong effort should be made to provide various technological aids that can widen the vocational horizons of the blind.

To implement the program we propose three specific actions:

1. A committee on sensory aids, providing connective structure among federal agencies and scientific and technical communities. A suggested vehicle is the National Academy of Sciences/National Academy of Engineering/National Research Council, since that organization is well placed to recruit advisory panels who can formulate long-range plans, review proposals, and advise on funding.

2. An information center on blindness, providing a primary channel for dissemination of information to workers, users, and other interested individuals. Suggested responsible agencies are the National Institute for Neurological Diseases and Blindness and the American Foundation for the Blind.

3. Several research centers combining the mutually beneficial resources of university and industrial organizations capable of making contributions to fundamental and applied research and development.

This report results from the discussions at a meeting of the subcommittee on sensory aids of the Committee on Prosthetics Research and Development held at the National Academy of Sciences in Washington, D.C., on 30 and 31 March, 1967.

Appendix 6:
EXCERPT FROM "REPORT FOR RESEARCH ON SENSORY AIDS FOR THE DEAF"

INTRODUCTION

The purpose of this report is to outline the problems of providing sensory aids for the deaf and to indicate the present status and future requirements of related research.

There are several profound distinctions between the problems of the deaf and those of the blind, resulting in significant differences in sensory aid research and in the training of the handicapped. These distinctions are due to the combined effect of two factors: man's ability for abstract thinking depends greatly on his capacity for acquiring and using language, and the acquisition of speech and language is strongly associated with the ability to hear. The deaf, therefore, require sensory aids not only to facilitate their communication with others—as do the blind—but also to acquire language.

It follows that the use of sensory aids for the deaf presents two separate problems may require different approaches. Those who became deaf *after* acquiring language may need education only in the use of a sensory aid. Those who were born deaf or who became deaf very early will require additional sensory aids for language acquisition. Further, there are severe problems of speech production as well as speech acquisition. These problems are important to a relatively large proportion of our population.

Modern technology provides a variety of sensory aid devices for the deaf. The operating principles are either to give as much useful sound amplification as possible, using whatever residual hearing the deaf may have or to detect and transform certain acoustic features into signals in other sensory modalities. However, while the essential technology for such devices is well established, the merit of these devices has not been fully evaluated, and optimum methods for using them or for training users are largely unknown.

In this report, therefore, existing technology as well

as future technological possibilities will be summarized, and principal stress will be placed on required research for finding the best methods of utilizing existing sensory aids, on finding optimum methods of teaching, on teacher training, and on methods of device and system evaluation.

Though adequate hearing implies a great variety of perceived sounds, speech, because of its overwhelming importance, will receive greatest emphasis. Although the primary stress will be on devising useful sensory aids, this goal implies underlying and related interests which are much broader in scope. Practically all research in sensory communication impinges in some way on the specific objectives for deaf communication. In particular, research findings in physiological and psychological acoustics suggest new and sophisticated possibilities for diagnosis of hearing problems. Similarly, perceptual measurements on synthetic and processed speech suggest design criteria for communication aids. Research in these and related areas must be followed closely and turned to advantage where possible in establishing techniques and aids for deaf communication.

PRESENT STATUS

As pointed out in the Introduction, two kinds of sensory aids are available for the deaf: one type concentrates on optimum ways of sound amplification, while the other attempts some kind of signal transformation, usually into another sensory modality.

Task Group Report on Skeletal Prostheses and Neuromuscular Control

Melvin J. Glimcher
EDITH M. ASHLEY PROFESSOR OF ORTHOPEDIC SURGERY
MASSACHUSETTS GENERAL HOSPITAL, CO-CHAIRMAN

Robert W. Mann
PROFESSOR OF MECHANICAL ENGINEERING
MASSACHUSETTS INSTITUTE OF TECHNOLOGY, CO-CHAIRMAN

Dr. Alan Cudworth
DIRECTOR, LIBERTY MUTUAL RESEARCH CENTER
HOPKINTON, MASSACHUSETTS

William H. Harris
ASSOCIATE ORTHOPEDIC SURGEON
MASSACHUSETTS GENERAL HOSPITAL

Robert M. Kenedi
MECHANICAL ENGINEERING DEPARTMENT
STRATHCLYDE UNIVERSITY
GLASGOW, SCOTLAND

Jacob L. Meiry
ASSISTANT PROFESSOR OF AERONAUTICS
MASSACHUSETTS INSTITUTE OF TECHNOLOGY

James B. Morrison
RESEARCH ASSOCIATE IN MECHANICAL ENGINEERING
MASSACHUSETTS INSTITUTE OF TECHNOLOGY

Igor Paul
ASSISTANT PROFESSOR OF MECHANICAL ENGINEERING
MASSACHUSETTS INSTITUTE OF TECHNOLOGY

Donald S. Pierce
ASSISTANT ORTHOPEDIC SURGEON
MASSACHUSETTS GENERAL HOSPITAL

Charles Radcliffe
DEPARTMENT OF MECHANICAL ENGINEERING
BIOMECHANICS LABORATORY
UNIVERSITY OF CALIFORNIA, BERKELEY

Eric L. Radin
RESEARCH FELLOW IN ORTHOPEDIC SURGERY
MASSACHUSETTS GENERAL HOSPITAL

Robert M. Rose
ASSOCIATE PROFESSOR OF METALLURGY
MASSACHUSETTS INSTITUTE OF TECHNOLOGY

Kenneth A. Smith
ASSOCIATE PROFESSOR OF CHEMICAL ENGINEERING
MASSACHUSETTS INSTITUTE OF TECHNOLOGY

Daniel E. Whitney
ASSISTANT PROFESSOR OF MECHANICAL ENGINEERING
MASSACHUSETTS INSTITUTE OF TECHNOLOGY

Laurence R. Young
ASSOCIATE PROFESSOR OF AERONAUTICS
MASSACHUSETTS INSTITUTE OF TECHNOLOGY

Collaboration between M.I.T. faculty and Harvard Medical School-Massachusetts General Hospital orthopedic surgeons has extended over ten years and currently includes M.I.T. Professors Mann, Paul, and Whitney from mechanical engineering, Professors Young and Meiry from aeronautics & astronautics, and Drs. Glimcher, Harris, Pierce, DeLorme, and Radin from the Harvard Medical School faculty. Biomechanical projects have benefited from the research and rehabilitation staffs and facilities support of the Liberty Mutual Insurance Company, which has also augmented fiscal support from federal agencies and private foundations.

Shared experiences in biomedical engineering research, development, and evaluation projects currently include:

1. an electromyographically controlled artificial limb approaching clinical prescription (Appendix 1);
2. determination of the temporal and spatial pressure distribution across the human hip joint (Appendix 2);
3. biomechanical and biochemical studies of joint function, lubrication and wear (Appendix 3);
4. the study of postural control and the microphysiology of skeletal muscles (Appendix 4); and
5. design of braces and mobility assisting devices.

Professor Rose and his colleagues in the Metallurgy Department at MIT have underway electrochemical corrosion studies directed toward the development of ultra-resistant alloys and non-metals for human implantation.

Professor Smith's studies of the chemistry of the synovial fluid is directly relevant to the joint lubrication investigation.

Opportunities

More formal organizational lines, closer geographical contiguity, certain essential and desirable facilities, and adequate supportive staff would accelerate and fructify existing projects by synergistically interweaving interests and efforts. Pending and prospective efforts would greatly benefit from more intimate interaction. Examples of such potential interaction include: single muscle fibre and individual motor unit microelectrode studies of myopathic and neuropathic diseases entities and spasticity underway at Massachusetts General Hospital in relation to a recently defined Sc.D. thesis on signla detection and of information processing from peripheral nerve bundles as the source of direct volitional control of prostheses; the biological applications of ultracorrosion resistant alloys and nonmetals; the control of multi-degree-of-freedom artificial limbs in relation to research on tele-operators and human augmentation; human sensory system studies undertaken for man-vehicle control purposes in relation to enhancement of sensory feedback from artificial limbs to the amputee; the application of knowledge in mechanical kinematics, friction and lubrication, strength of materials, and structures to the design, evaluation, and application of more effective body and limb braces and external and internal body prostheses.

Resources

Our primary goal is to apply and reinforce the basic resources of engineering talent at M.I.T. and medical strength of Harvard Medical School-Massachusetts General Hospital to realize tangible benefits to physically impaired people and extend that knowledge essential to alleviating human infirmity.

Our resources are:

1. the respective university and hospital faculties;
2. graduate students in both engineering and medicine who have elected to pursue a biological-medical-engineering education and to undertake with the faculty the research of enhanced knowledge and the design of improved means for human rehabilitation;
3. the physical facilities, staff, and very important, the patients of the hospital; and
4. the special facilities and staff support at the Institute.

We recognize that biomedical engineering is a team effort to be shaped among the medical, engineering, and the physical sciences. These faculty orientations and the substantial education prerequisites of both areas demand organizational and physical arrangements that encourage and produce close, continuous interaction. Since our product, be it hardware or knowledge, is intrinsically people-centered, close contact with the patients is also essential.

Recommendations

We make interlocking recommendations to realize these opportunities in the spirit of the NAE–NIH study for prototypes of bioengineering activity and in recognition of Harvard–M.I.T. studies of engineering and living systems collaboration. Given the locations of the Institute, Harvard Medical School, and Massachusetts General Hospital, the essential access to patients, the familiarity of engineers with the hospital and medical personnel with engineering research, design and developmental environment, in order to provide space and facilities to carry through the goals in biomechanics, we recommend a biomechanical group in a bioengineering center (preferably located between Massachusetts General Hospital and M.I.T.) and a biomechanics research and development facility as part of the rehabilitation unit at Massachusetts General Hospital.

The Massachusetts General Hospital Rehabilitation Unit

The rehabilitation unit in White 9 and North 9 at Massachusetts General Hospital will include fifty-six beds, physical and occupational therapy, and an electromyograph lab. The rehabilitation clinic (1,000 square feet) will be in North 1, with a large brace and prosthetics shop below in the basement with at least one research prosthetist and one research orthotist. Application has been made to the hospital's space committee for an additional 3,000 square feet of the sub-basement directly under the brace shop, which we propose as the biomechanics research and development facility. This facility would have office space for a faculty member and several research assistants from engineering as well as laboratory facilities. This hospital location would provide direct access to patient-related studies being conducted in the hospital's rehabilitation unit and clinic.

The Bioengineering Center

The biomechanics group in the bioengineering center would be research and development oriented. Office space for perhaps six faculty (both engineering faculty and medical doctors) would provide supervision for perhaps ten to fifteen graduate assistants conducting masters and doctoral level investigations.

In turn the biomechanics group would be one of several such divisions of the bioengineering center, each having access to and sharing common center facilities, which would include: equipment and supporting staff; a specialized library; seminar rooms; analog, digital, and hybrid computation; animal care facilities; operating rooms; tissue and culture preparation labs; shielded biotelemetry rooms with provision for synchronized bi- and tri-planer photography; electron microscope, electron beam and micro-probe, neutron activation analysis, X-ray, fluoroscopy, and defraction facilities; instrument rooms, and machine shops.

The physical design of the bioengineering center must provide for clinical cleanliness, chemical cleanliness, and electro-magnetic shielding of experimental space which will include operating rooms.

The Development and Evaluation Process

The bioengineering center must also identify itself with and assume responsibility for the engineering development and the human evaluation of devices and prostheses initiated by its staff. One of the major national problems in the application of technology to biological and medical applications is the problem of transition from research and first-feasibility demonstration in an academic or medical environment, by means of engineering development and evaluation that test the efficacy of the design on reasonable-sized and representative populations, leading ultimately to the manufacture and deployment to practitioners in the field and their patients. The traditional academic grouping of faculty supervisor and graduate student (with very modest engineering and technical back-up) produces successful feasibility demonstrations, but redesign is inevitable in order to produce small lots of reliable, reproducible entities for first small-scale evaluation and, subsequently, field and clinical testing. In our free-enterprise, consumer economy, this process of redesign for production and consumer evaluation is borne by the manufacturer as part of his production costs and is reflected in small per-unit increases in the final price of the commodity. Where large volume production and distribution is anticipated, these developmental and evaluation costs prove manageable. Moreover, in most complex products a process of design evolution goes on, with new offerings representing minor changes in established lines.

Biomedical engineering has not yet undergone the historical evolution that permits evaluation; assessment is further complicated by the product's direct and potentially serious influence on patients' health and well-being; and with no surveyable markets or distribution systems there has been as yet no substantial commitment of venture capital searching for large volume sales. If the bioengineering center is to effect significant contributions to human welfare it must at the outset assume responsibility for development and evaluation. Admittedly, costs in this area are generally of greater magnitude than investments in the usual faculty-supervised graduate student research and feasibility demonstration of a new approach. However, while developmental capability must not inhibit original contributions, a full-time developmental staff of any size can handle only a small portion of the projects being explored by the faculty-graduate student teams, so the most rigorous scrutiny must apply to the choice of projects slated for development and evaluation.

The bioengineering center will certainly require an advisory committee that is intimately informed on the various studies underway, so they can decide which candidates warrant the large investment of staff and resources necessary for subsequent development and evaluation.

The staff of the center ought to establish connections with many manufacturing, distribution, and evaluation resources that can assist the process of development and evaluation. Devices that lend themselves to external development should be exploited: evaluation could occur in the hospital, the clinic, or the community. Under any circumstances, the management of the center must recognize the vital importance of assuming responsibility for ultimate deployment but at the same time maintain great flexibility in the ways in which this deployment might be achieved.

A Prototype of Collaboration with Industry

The experience of M.I.T., Harvard Medical School, and Massachusetts General Hospital with Liberty Mutual Insurance Company provides a prototype of how the academic base of biomedical development and evaluation can be extended. The basic work leading to the present electromyographically controlled limb (Appendix 1) was undertaken in the academic departments of electrical and mechanical engineering at the institute in the context of faculty-supervised, graduate student theses. From the outset the program was, in part, supported by the Liberty Mutual Insurance Company, which supplemented research contract support from the Vocational Rehabilitation Administration of the Department of Health, Education & Welfare. Student theses having demonstrated the feasibility of the concept, the problem of how to extend the project to hardware that could be evaluated on amputees became apparent. Liberty Mutual was responsive to the proposal of Professor Mann that it retain the services of full-time experienced, electronic and mechanical design engineers to conduct the development and redesign, and it assumed the financial responsibility and provided an appropriate environment for the professional engineers in its research center in Hopkinton, Massachusetts.

The prothesis project has been subsequently supervised by an orthopedic surgeon, engineering professor team, with contributions from Liberty's research center director and from the staff of the company's rehabilitation center in Boston, which is now conducting the fittings and evaluations of the limb. Clinical prescritpion is anticipated, although the question of ultimate manufacture and distribution is not yet resolved.

Participation from Management

Given the crucial nature of this problem of transfer from research feasibility through development and evaluation into deployment in the field, the bioengineering center should be of interest to faculty and students concerned with research, development, evaluation, and deployment per se, including questions such as industrial organization, administration, market development, and distribution. The Sloan School of Industrial Management and Harvard Business School faculty should be invited to participate and make contributions. A modest example of a specific study of the impact of new technology on braille production was recently sponsored by the Mechanical Engineering Group on Sensory Aids.[1]

Staff

Organization and physical arrangements of the center and the research group at the rehabilitation facility must emphasize the collaborative nature of biomedical engineering. Both buildings must provide offices for engineering and medical faculty, though in most cases they will not all be present at either location. Names on doors and desk or lab space will encourage the engineering faculty to spend time at the hospital and medical staff at the bioengineering center. Organizational arrangements should provide joint appointments in the engineering school and medical school or hospital for those who participate.

Long-term staffing in bioengineering activity will be only partially resolved by joint appointments, however. In most cases these serve to supplement an already established base of professional competence and only indirectly affect the prospect of promotion and tenure. While a joint appointment for an engineering faculty person will significantly supplement his effectiveness in bioengineering work, his main center of activity and advancement will remain his department and the school of engineering. Similarly, Harvard faculty jointly appointed at the institute would simply be supplementing a prime base.

Considering the autonomy of the institutions involved and their own priorities, it may be naive to assume that the urgency of appointment of, say, medically based people will be shared by the medical institution. There is already evidence that personnel specializing in physical-based science and holding appointments in the medical institution experience advancement difficulties in the medically oriented environment. In any case, the institutions themselves must devise organizational accommodations for appointments and promotions.

External Advice

The task group benefited substantially from the experiences of a faculty member of the University of California Biomechanics Laboratory, which has been in existence since the end of World War II, and from the director of the Bioengineering Institute at the University of Strathclyde in Glasgow (Appendix 5).

They advised us on problems of organization, interdisciplinary collaboration, research, development, evaluation and deployment and the difficulties of establishing priorities, the absolute necessity of intimate patient interaction, the need to strike reasonable balances between different approaches, and much more modest but realizable engineering and medical contributions, for example, of the problem of "deskilling" devices and prostheses in order to make them applicable to large-scale populations of practitioners and clients. Problems of bioengineering are refreshingly similar, whether approached on the east and west coasts of this nation or in Europe.

[1] L. H. Goldish, "Braille in the United States: Its Production, Distribution and Use." Thesis (S.M.), Sloan School of Management, Massachusetts Institute of Technology, February 1967. (Also published as a State-of-the-Art Report by the American Foundation for the Blind, New York City, December 1967).

Appendix 1: Design Criteria, Development and Pre- and Post-Fitting Amputee Evaluation of an EMG Controlled, Force Sensing, Proportional-Rate, Elbow Prosthesis with Cutaneous Kinesthetic Feedback

ROBERT W. MANN

ABSTRACT

Cybernetical research and development has resulted in a prosthesis for above-elbow amputees that is controlled in a continuous and graded manner by the surface detection of electrical potentials generated by neuromuscular activity in the otherwise nonfunctional residual muscles in the amputee's stump. The rate of rotation of the forearm or the force at the terminal device is related to the amputee's conscious effort. The limb's servosystem also senses terminal load and adjusts gain accordingly. Research has demonstrated the feasibility of introducing kinesthetic feedback of elbow angle to the amputee by means of a cutaneous, phantomsensation presentation on the upper arm stump. All mechanical and electronic components are integrated into an otherwise cosmetic forearm with power provided by a belt-mounted battery pack. Initial determination of the limb's mechanical and electrical characteristics was established by means of computer simulation. The testing of normal and amputee subjects on a simulated tracking task has evaluated their comparative EMG control potentials. Satisfactory conscious control of the artificial limb has been achieved within five minutes after fitting on an amputee. A small lot of prototype limbs will undergo laboratory evaluation, clinical testing, then everyday use.

Appendix 2:
ABSTRACT FROM DOCTORAL THESIS, "MEASUREMENT OF PRESSURE DISTRIBUTION IN THE HUMAN HIP JOINT"

CHARLES E. CARBON
DEPARTMENT OF MECHANICAL ENGINEERING
MASSACHUSETTS INSTITUTE OF TECHNOLOGY

GOAL

The object of the proposed investigation is to measure directly the spatial and temporal pressure distribution on articular cartilage surfaces in the normal human hip joint. The pressure distribution will be measured for such activities as walking, stair climbing, and single-leg support.

MOTIVATION

The human hip joint is a subject of interest in several research areas. Wear patterns (areas of well-defined cartilage deterioration) have been observed in damaged or diseased hip joints. Direct measurement of the pressure distribution would help determine the correlation between pressure and cartilage wear or disease. The lubricating mechanism between the articular cartilage surfaces is poorly understood, and a knowledge of the pressure distribution between the sliding surfaces in the hip joint would contribute to a better understanding of joint mechanics and human gait. Knowledge of the pressure distribution would also be of use to designers of prosthetic devices.

References

1. Verne T. Inman, "Functional Aspects of the Abductor Muscles of the Hip," *The Journal of Bone and Joint Surgery*, 29 (July 1947) : 607–619.

2. J. P. Paul, "Forces Transmitted by Joints in the Human Body," *Symposium on Lubrication and Wear in Living and Artificial Human Joints* (London: Institution of Mechanical Engineers, 1967).

3. Nils W. Rydell, *Forces Acting on the Femoral Head-Prosthesis*. Goteborg (Sweden: Tryckeri AB Litotyp, 1966).

4. Charles E. Carlson, "Measurement of Pressure Distribution in the Human Hip Joint." SM. thesis, Massachusetts Institute of Technology, 1967.

Appendix 3: Wear and Friction in Animal Joints

IGOR PAUL
ERIC RADIN

The Mechanical Engineering Department at M.I.T. and the orthopedic research laboratories at the Massachusetts General Hospital have already embarked on a long-term collaborative effort in the area of joint physiology. This work is directed towards a better understanding of the physical behavior of joints and the contributions of various joint components (i.e., joint synovial fluid, cartilage and subchondral bone) on this behavior.

Some work on the frictional properties of animal joints had previously been completed by Dr. Radin and reported in the literature. A comprehensive research plan was developed from this work in conjunction with the mechanical engineering department at M.I.T.

Work has already begun on defining the mechanical properties of articular cartilage, joint fluid, and underlying bone. Methods have been devised to measure impact forces and coefficients of friction of loaded joints. Long-term studies of wear, as well as measurements of the mechanical behavior of joints that have been treated to alter their physical properties, will be carried out.

The collaboration of medical and engineering disciplines in this clearly interdisciplinary area of research has been found to be extremely desirable since the understanding and measurements of the lubrication and wear processes in joints is dependent on basic engineering principles as well as on medical considerations.

It is hoped that this collaboration will be expanded to include the departments of material sciences and chemical engineering at M.I.T. and to involve orthopedic research fellows and Harvard and M.I.T. students in this project.

The implications of the information derived from this work are obvious both in the treatment and prevention of arthritis in man and in the design of joint replacements.

Appendix 4: Studies of Human Dynamic Space Orientation Using Techniques of Control Theory

L. R. YOUNG AND Y.T. LI
MAN—VEHICLE LABORATORY
CENTER FOR SPACE RESEARCH
MASSACHUSETTS INSTITUTE OF TECHNOLOGY

POSTURAL AND NEUROMUSCULAR CONTROL

With increasing amounts of quantitative physiological data on neuromuscular control becoming available, a "rational parameter" approach to understanding the "neuromuscular lag" component of the human operator describing function appears reasonable. Some interesting new neuromuscular models have been reported, and two projects are being carried out in our laboratory. One of these is a new attempt to create a neuromuscular model based on "component models" for triple muscle innervation (two gammas and one alpha), dual afferents (stretch and stretch rate), Golgi tendon organs, joint receptors, and Renshaw cells. John Allum plans to apply control theory to the problem of analyzing the alpha and gamma stimulation loops. The other project is an input-output, using postural control as an example. The following summary is from the Ph.D. thesis proposal of Lewis Nashner.

The goal of this thesis is to model the flow and interaction of sensory information necessary for man to maintain posture. Formulating a model of posture control directly from physiology would be difficult for several reasons.

1. A complete description of the neural circuitry involved in posture control is not known.

2. Experimental observation of the many information channels in man is not practical.

Instead of being a necessarily weak model, based on neurophysiological data, the model will be developed by defining two major posture control modes. After a thorough experimental description of these two control modes, the resulting model will be reexamined in the light of current physiological evidence.

The reflex response is defined as a continuous linear control of limb position and force output, responding to muscle length and tension only. The response will have terms proportional to displacement and to the rate of displacement. The gains of the length and velocity terms are independently variable over a limited range.

The orienting response is defined as the control of posture with respect to the external environment. The orienting control responds to proprioceptor, visual, and motion cues. The response reflects both subconscious learned patterns and the conscious desires of the man. Because the orienting response incorporates complex processing patterns and memory, its output can be expected to be of significantly different form from that of the reflex response.

Since the passive dynamic characteristics of the body and its reflex responses have common variables, the total dynamic characteristics of the body will be viewed as the combination of these properties. The control of the reflex response "gains" is therefore a parametric control of the body's dynamic characteristics. The other inputs are the external disturbances and the orienting responses. From this viewpoint posture control is effected in two ways:

1. with orienting responses, reacting to the body's motions in respect to its external environment; and

2. with the parametric control of the body's dynamic characteristics, both to orienting response commands and to external disturbances.

A major emphasis of the model will be a description of the relative roles of the two posture control modes. The total range of the reflex response control of the body's dynamic characteristics will be determined experimentally. The criteria by which control is delegated between the two modes for a variety of external conditions will be described.

Appendix 5:
FINAL REPORT ON THE BIOMECHANICS RESEARCH GROUP, 1963–1967 UNIVERSITY OF STRATHCLYDE GLASGOW

Contents

Task Group Report on Subcellular Engineering

D. Michael Young
ASSISTANT PROFESSOR OF BIOLOGICAL CHEMISTRY
HARVARD MEDICAL SCHOOL, CHAIRMAN

Howard C. Berg
ASSISTANT PROFESSOR OF BIOLOGY AND CHAIRMAN OF THE BOARD OF
TUTORS IN BIOCHEMICAL SCIENCES
HARVARD UNIVERSITY

Joseph D. Fleming
INSTRUMENTATION LAB
MASSACHUSETTS INSTITUTE OF TECHNOLOGY

John Gilbert
STAFF STATISTICIAN
HARVARD COMPUTING CENTER

Jerome Gross
ASSOCIATE PROFESSOR OF MEDICINE
MASSACHUSETTS GENERAL HOSPITAL

Edgar Haber
ASSISTANT PROFESSOR OF MEDICINE
DEPARTMENT OF CARDIOLOGY
MASSACHUSETTS GENERAL HOSPITAL

Paul R. Schimmel
ASSISTANT PROFESSOR OF CHEMISTRY AND BIOLOGY
MASSACHUSETTS INSTITUTE OF TECHNOLOGY

The subcommittee on subcellular engineering met at the Faculty Club of the Massachusetts Institute of Technology on July 2 and 9, 1968. The committee was charged with the following responsibilities: (1) to consider ways in which engineering and biology might merge together in profitable research activities at the subcellular level; (2) to identify problem areas that would promote more effective interplay between engineering and basic biological research; and (3) to propose an appropriate organizational framework within which collaborative efforts between engineering and biology might flourish.

The Scope of Subcellular Engineering

Initially, the committee examined the meaning and scope of subcellular engineering. This discipline is a broad one, but it seemed to most that it largely encompassed biophysics, biochemistry and molecular biology. This report examines ways in which biophysicists, biochemists and molecular biologists can structure effective interplay with the engineering sciences.

The substance of the committee's discussions focused mainly upon two areas: ways in which the engineering sciences might bear more heavily upon the instrumentation problems that biologists face in their laboratories; and areas in which biologists can collaborate meaningfully with engineers in creative research.

Engineering Technology and Instrumentation in Biological Research

By its nature, molecular biology is not primarily an instrument- or machine-oriented science. Most biochemists, for example, are not primarily concerned with electronic instrumentation for its own sake. On the other hand, there are few natural sciences that rely more heavily upon sophisticated laboratory equipment than does fundamental biology. Thus, throughout their careers most biologists will often find themselves either tinkering with a piece of equipment to solve a new problem or in need of the design and construction of sophisticated and commercially unavailable new instruments.

The committee believes that technical assistance from

engineering personnel would be of great value in the area of instrumentation related to biological research. At present, one problem is simply that most biologists frequently feel incompetent to identify appropriate engineering talent when faced with technical problems beyond their competence. As an example, let us consider the problem of the design of a relatively sophisticated piece of electronic equipment, such as a special interface that would allow a laboratory instrument to be compatible with a digital computer. This is the kind of problem that a biologist can define readily in his own laboratory. Yet it is also a problem that he is probably ill-suited to solve. Solutions to some of these problems can indeed be implemented within the framework of good machine or electronic shops plus computer consulting services, but a good many require advanced engineering knowledge.

At the present time, it would appear that research and development of this kind is hampered by biologists' inability to find appropriate engineering personnel to whom they could turn for assistance. Several possible solutions to this problem were discussed, and the committee believes that a directory of personnel in the engineering sciences could play a useful role. Such a directory could take several forms. It would be helpful simply to have available a list of members of an engineering faculty who might welcome a consulative or collaborative role with their colleagues in biology. In conjunction with the directory, a liaison office might be established to foster free access between biology and engineering. It might also make available information of interest to both groups. A steering committee of engineers and biologists might implement such an office.

To give an example of how such an arrangement might work, let us suppose that a biological investigator is in need of assistance in the design of a new optical system. It would be the function of the liaison office to aid in contacting interested members of an engineering faculty who could not only provide the necessary knowledge, but might also wish to participate actively in a developmental project.

We have enumerated several examples of important instrumentation problems in molecular biology whose solution would be of value and which could provide a common meeting ground for the biological and engineering sciences.

1. ANALYTICAL TECHNIQUES IN BIOCHEMISTRY

Amino Acids analyses and amino acid and nucleic synthesis techniques are playing an ever widening role in biochemistry. Much of the success in elucidating the structures of complex macromolecules has stemmed from instrumentation developments in analysis techniques. It is clear that increasing degrees of automation of these analytical procedures can both enhance the accuracy of measurement and reduce direct operator time significantly. For example, it would be useful to have means available for automatic sample injection as well as computer monitoring of output from such machines. Moreover, one of the problems involved in work of this kind involves the type of ion-exchange resin employed. Advances in chemistry and chemical engineering in developing new resins and separation techniques could considerably advance the art of analytical biochemistry.

2. IMAGE PROCESSING TECHNIQUES

Image processing research will undoubtedly play an increasing role in identifying and characterizing cellular systems. This technique, now in its infancy, could be used, in principle, to measure and locate within a cell specific structures in a statistically significant sample and to validly describe experimental changes in specific cell populations. In tissue culture, for example, it might be possible to map and evaluate the mechanisms whereby cells adhere to one another and the patterns within which they grow.

3. SEPARATION TECHNIQUES AT THE CELLULAR AND SUBCELLULAR LEVEL

One of the principal problems involved in sorting out the complexities of a cellular system involves identification and separation of subcellular organelles and substances. In most cases at present, separation and preparation of these particles must be tediously carried out on a small scale. We believe that better ways could be sought to isolate and store these cell materials on a larger scale. It may be that the separation of whole living cells from a tissue into homogeneous species will become a problem of major importance.

4. ELECTRON MICROSCOPY AND ITS APPLICATIONS

The power of the electron microscope in biological research is enormous. Advances over the last decade have now made it possible to visualize not only viruses and bacteria, but also macromolecules of biological interest. Of the several technical problems in electron microscopy, one that has received insufficient attention is the support structure used for preparing specimens. The microscopist's aim in high-resolution work with macromolecules is to achieve the greatest signal-to-noise ratio possible, and in many cases, particularly where shadowing is used, resolution is limited by the support film. If ways could be found to prepare thin films with suitable surface properties, it should be possible to extend the limit of resolution for biological materials to previously unobtainable levels. Carbon and mica substrates have been used for this purpose, but the development of thin film techniques could well provide a new avenue of approach. Little work has been done to apply thin film techniques to microscopy, and this could be a problem that would interest chemical engineers.

5. MICROSPECTROPHOTOMETRY

It seems probable that one of the important developments in the future of cell research will be the use of spectrophotometric techniques in the analysis of individual living cells and their constituents *in situ*. Although much effort has been devoted in the past to these methods, particularly by Caspersson in Sweden, Uretz in Chicago, and others, there remain serious limitations. One problem is that appropriate high-sensitivity sensing devices combined with low-intensity radiation sources have not been developed to satisfactory levels. It is reasonable to assume that whereas sophisticated photomultiplication techniques have been widely used in astronomy, such devices might be adapted for analysis of the location of organelles within cells as well as for analysis of cell movement. Much of our knowledge of the substructure of cellular systems has arisen from biochemical information. Yet this very information has been derived primarily from bits and pieces of cells following their destruction. It seems clear in the future that we shall want to study and describe the anatomy and function of the cell and its components as they exist in the native, intact state, with minimum interference from the probe.

6. THE PROBLEM OF THE "UNIQUE" INSTRUMENT

In many areas of biological research, there is a prominent need for engineering know-how in the design of equipment that is commercially unavailable and has application only for a specific problem. Not infrequently, instrumental design of this kind suffers from a lack of appropriate engineering support and the fact that the biologist is by training unable to provide an electronic or machine shop with the necessary design information. Collaboration between engineers and biologists could go a long way in removing this barrier.

The Engineering Sciences and Fundamental Research in Subcellular Biology

The information presented above provides a few examples of feasible technological problems that engineers and biologists could profitably attack in collaborative work. The committee also recognized that one of its tasks was to consider a more fundamental problem relating to the direct collaboration of engineers and biologists in creative biological research. We have considered this problem carefully and should like to summarize our discussions of the question of what kind of conceptual interplay is feasible between biologists and engineers.

The topic provoked considerable discussion since it was particulary difficult to identify clear-cut problems or areas in molecular biology that could inspire creative conceptual thinking among engineers. In particular, it was pointed out that the training of biologists (indeed the language of biology) is substantially different from that encountered in engineering. Consequently, the committee suggested that education of individuals both in engineering and the biological sciences might be a necessary prerequisite for meaningful collaborative research among these two groups. We recognize that another task group committee is evaluating the problem of biomedical engineering curricula, but the problems of research and education are clearly interdependent. Several members of the committee, including both engineers and biologists, felt that meaningful collaborative research between two quite different disciplines depends upon a mutual understanding by both kinds of scientists of the nature of that discipline. Thus, if we are to structure a useful common ground for collaborative research, both biologists and engineers might necessarily require broad experience in two fields. Problems in molecular biology and biochemistry, as in any other science, arise largely from ideas generated in individual laboratories by biologists doing biology. At the present time, the committee seriously wondered how often new ideas would arise from the engineering sciences until engineers have been sufficiently trained at the graduate level in a biological discipline. The committee wishes to make clear that this dilemma, if it truly exists, may well be unique to fundamental biology as opposed to applied research in the medical sciences where problems are more clearly identifiable and solutions more easily recognizable.

The sense of this committee is that the growth and advancement of basic biology stems almost entirely from pursuit of basic concepts. Insofar as subcellular biology is concerned, it would appear to remain for biologists to continue to identify problems of importance, and further, that the engineering sciences might not be able at this time to participate broadly in biological research. For these reasons, the Committee favors training interested and motivated individuals in a multidisciplinary way as a meaningful first step to fostering an interplay between engineering and biology.

With these ideas in mind, the committee turned its attention to identifying some of the major conceptual problems now facing biological scientists.

1. THE SELF-ASSEMBLY OF CELLULAR AND ORGANIC SYSTEMS

At the present time, much of our understanding of the way genes act, as well as our knowledge of the structure and function of macromolecules, indicates that the day may be near when biologists understand the forces responsible for ordering of cellular systems. For example, what is it that makes an arm an arm, and a liver a liver, and how might we begin to use first principles in biology to understand how these unique structures are assembled? This is a major problem in embryological research, and it underlies the problem of regeneration in biological systems. It was not clear to the committee just how the engineering sciences might participate in this activity.

2. INFORMATION STORAGE AND THE BASIS OF MEMORY

Much of our knowledge in this area stems from information on the physiological properties of neural systems. Neurophysiology and electrophysiology have contributed to our understanding of conduction processes in nerve cells, and the engineering sciences have contributed to the instrumentation used in this highly specialized field. Although it is difficult to predict what direction future studies will take, it seems clear to us that an understanding of control systems and information theory will be of significant value in formulating suitable experiments to unravel the memory storage problem. Nevertheless, it is difficult for biologists to think of feasible ways in which a chemical information storage system could operate. Again, this is probably an area that will receive its greatest impetus from an idea or concept generated in an individual research laboratory.

3. COMPUTER SIMULATION TECHNIQUES

It has only been in the past few years that the computer has found its way into biological research. This development has been important not only for the more straightforward problems of data storage and retrieval but also for simulation of macromolecular structure, metabolic pathways and biological control mechanisms. Newer techniques in image processing and pattern recognition could be of great value to the biologist, not only in the designing of appropriate experiments but also in the visual display of experimental parameters. The computer display of macromolecular structure has already received significant attention, and it is likely that an extension of these techniques to other areas of cellular biology would be of value.

4. BIOLOGICAL ENERGETICS

Our understanding of biochemical energetics now allows us to formulate in concrete terms several of the ways in which energy transformations occur in living systems. The committee feels that much of this information could be brought to bear upon the problem of powering artificial devices such as a mechanical heart pump. Solutions to this problem (were it feasible) must stem from an understanding of the appropriate energy-producing pathways of the cells as well as the electrochemical basis of energy transformations.

5. INTERCELLULAR COMMUNICATION MECHANISMS

Most cells in living systems exist as tissue aggregates, and often the biological operation of each tissue is not just the arithmetic sum of its cellular component parts. Thus, cells communicate with one another, transport substances among themselves, and adhere in specialized, recognizable patterns. Undoubtedly, many of these cell characteristics are dependent upon specific surface membrane properties that are poorly understood. It may well be that biologists could learn much from their engineering colleagues about the structure and function of semipermeable barriers from the standpoints of both their physical properties and their chemical structure.

6. PHYSIOLOGICAL MANIPULATION OF SINGLE CELLS

Recent biochemical studies have demonstrated that the function and structure of macromolecules depends strongly upon their environment. We would expect that the macrostructure of a cell imposes constraints upon its various constituents that are not present when these components are observed separately. Thus, the mitochondrian as a cell organelle may function differently in its cellular environment than it does when observed *in vitro*. For systems of this kind, ways must be sought to examine and to alter the internal milieu of single cells. Such developments will undoubtedly require a new approach to the design and use of intracellular measuring devices as well as new techniques for stimulating cells and for recording their responses.

Organizational Framework

These observations reflect research areas that we believe could represent an appropriate foundation to foster closer interplay of biology with engineering. The committee has also considered the problem of the organizational framework under which this kind of collaboration could flourish. In the case of molecular biology, at least, the committee believed there would be few areas of overlap between biologists and engineers in which fruitful collaboration could be initiated except on an ad hoc basis. This feeling arises, from the concept that creative research, at least in biology, does not lend itself to multidisciplinary task force efforts. Truly new ideas in biology arise slowly, as in most other sciences; collaborative studies are not generated simply through individuals with diverse backgrounds being together. This is not to say that effective communication among biologists and engineers would not spur effective mutual collaboration. Indeed, we have tried to identify some of those areas in which joint efforts might be fruitful. On the other hand, the committee believes that a central framework whereby biologists and engineers would be thrown together under one roof is probably not appropriate at this time and indeed might prove disruptive. Thus, the rigid organizational framework of a multidisciplinary center would not be likely to foster a meaningful scientific program among biologists and engineers. This conclusion simply recognizes the fact that engineers and biologists are of two totally dissimilar disciplines, and effective long-term contacts would require long-term preparation by each. They may well have much to contribute to each other in the long run, but it seemed to the committee that developments for the near future at least should rest largely with the personal initiatives of both engineers and biologists to seek out and solve problems of interest to both, utilizing deliberately established and effective lines of communication. Within this experience, it might prove feasible to establish a more formal structure.

A Beginning

This book provides one approach to a university program in engineering and living systems. It is likely that as universities in this country and throughout the world embark on such programs that new ideas and local considerations will dictate changes in direction and detail and that other solutions may appear. Nevertheless, at this pioneering stage, we believe that this formulation in which disparate elements are interrelated does provide for a sound beginning.

Appendix:
CONFERENCE ON INTERACTIONS BETWEEN THE UNIVERSITY, INDUSTRIAL, AND MEDICAL CARE COMMUNITIES

Industrial Participants

Saul Aronow
CONSULTANT IN MEDICAL ENGINEERING
AMERICAN OPTICAL CORP., FRAMINGHAM, MASS.

Dr. H. J. Bixler
VICE-PRESIDENT—RESEARCH
AMICON CORP., LEXINGTON, MASS.

Dr. L. Blaney
MEDICAL DIRECTOR
SYLVANIA ELECTRONICS, WALTHAM, MASS.

Phillip R. Brooks
MANAGER OF DIGITAL SYSTEM RESEARCH
AMERICAN OPTICAL CORP., FRAMINGHAM, MASS.

Dr. Francis J. Bullock
SENIOR CHEMIST
ARTHUR D. LITTLE INC., CAMBRIDGE, MASS.

John D. Cann
ENGINEER
GRASS INSTRUMENT CO., QUINCY, MASS.

Robert A. Cross
ASSISTANT DIRECTOR OF RESEARCH
AMICON CORP., LEXINGTON, MASS.

Dr. T. B. Eyrick
E.G. & G. INC., BEDFORD, MASS.

Dr. Richard P. deFilippi
PROGRAM MANAGER
ABCOR INC., CAMBRIDGE, MASS.

Martin L. Fleischman
MEDICAL PRODUCT COORDINATOR
INSTRUMENTATION LABORATORY INC., WATERTOWN, MASS.

Dr. Tibor Foldvari
DIRECTOR OF RESEARCH AND DEVELOPMENT
HARVARD APPARATUS CO., MILLIS, MASS.

Hugo Freudenthal
MANAGER, LIFE SCIENCES
FAIRCHILD HILLER CORP., REPUBLIC AVIATION DIV., FARMINGDALE, N.Y.

Leon P. Gaucher
ASSISTANT TO MANAGER, SCIENTIFIC PLANNING
TEXACO INC., BEACON, N.Y.

Herbert Goldberg
MANAGER OF DEVELOPMENT AND ENGINEERING
AMERICAN OPTICAL CORP., BEDFORD, MASS.

Morton Goulder
CORPORATE SCIENTIST
SANDERS ASSOCIATES, NASHUA, N.H.

A. J. Gracia
VICE-PRESIDENT RESEARCH
GOODYEAR TIRE & RUBBER CO., AKRON, OHIO.

Dr. Gerry Guter
SECTION CHIEF, WATER TECHNOLOGY, ASTROPOWER LABORATORY
McDONNELL DOUGLAS AIRCRAFT CO., NEWPORT BEACH, CALIFORNIA.

Ihsan A. Haddad
MANAGER ENGINEERING CHEMISTRY
INSTRUMENTATION LABORATORY INC., WATERTOWN, MASS.

H. F. Halsted
MANAGER BIOCHEM. DIVISION
AEROJET GENERAL CORP., EL MONTE, CALIFORNIA.

Donald Hatfield
STAFF MEMBER
I.B.M. CORP., CAMBRIDGE, MASS.

H. Philip Hovnanian
MANAGER, BIOMEDICAL ENGINEERING DEPARTMENT
KOLLSMAN INSTRUMENT CORP., SYOSSET, L.I., N.Y.

Dr. Fred Huffman
SECTION MANAGER
THERMO ELECTRON CORP., WALTHAM, MASS.

Dr. Donald R. Johnson
RESEARCH & ENGINEERING MANAGER
E.I. DU PONT, INSTRUMENT PRODUCTS DIVISION, WILMINGTON, DELAWARE.

Dr. Arthur Kantrowitz
VICE-PRESIDENT
AVCO EVERETT RESEARCH LABORATORY, EVERETT, MASS.

Henry King
BIO-ENGINEERING CONSULTANT
HONEYWELL INC., BOSTON, MASS.

James F. Kistler
ENGINEERING SECTION MANAGER, MEDICAL INSTRUMENTS SECTION
HEWLETT-PACKARD CO., WALTHAM, MASS.

Charles J. Koester
APPLIED RESEARCH MANAGER
AMERICAN OPTICAL CORP., FRAMINGHAM CENTER, MASS.

Russell E. Long
GENERAL MANAGER, ENGINEERING & SYSTEMS DIVISION
ALLIED RESEARCH ASSOC. INC., CONCORD, MASS.

Ivan Lubash
MANAGER, PROGRAM DEVELOPMENT
SYLVANIA ELECTRONIC SYSTEMS, WALTHAM, MASS.

David Marshall
MEDICAL DIRECTOR
SANDERS ASSOCIATES, NASHUA, N.H.

Dr. Charles J. Martell
DIRECTOR, LIFE SCIENCES LABORATORY
NORTHROP CORP., HAWTHORNE, CALIFORNIA.

Dr. S. M. MacNeille
VICE-PRESIDENT & DIRECTOR OF RESEARCH
AMERICAN OPTICAL CORP., SOUTHBRIDGE, MASS.

John M. McIsaac, Jr.
PRODUCT MARKETING RESEARCH AND DEVELOPMENT
HAMILTON STANDARD DIVISION, UNITED AIRCRAFT, FARMINGTON, CONN.

Wm. Ralph Mercer
CORPORATE SCIENTIST
SANDERS ASSOCIATES INC., NASHUA, N.H.

Barry Moxon
MARKETING MANAGER
AEROJET GENERAL CORP., EL MONTE, CALIFORNIA.

Wm. Mullahy
TECHNICAL PRODUCTS
AMERICAN OPTICAL CORP., SOUTHBRIDGE, MASS.

Frank Paolini
SENIOR SCIENTIST
AMERICAN SCIENCE & ENGINEERING INC., CAMBRIDGE, MASS.

Dr. Henry G. Pars
HEAD, MEDICAL CHEMISTRY
ARTHUR D. LITTLE INC., CAMBRIDGE, MASS.

R. M. Pierson
MANAGER, SYNTHETIC RUBBER RESEARCH
GOODYEAR TIRE & RUBBER CO., AKRON, OHIO

Edward J. Poitras
DIRECTOR OF ENGINEERING
FENWAL INC., ASHLAND, MASS.

A. Rasiel
GENERAL MANAGER, BIO-ENGINEERING
E.G. & G., SALEM, MASS.

Tom Roberts
MANAGER, HEALTH PRODUCTS
BORG-WARNER, DES PLAINES, ILLINOIS

Thomas Robinson
SECTION MANAGER
THERMO ELECTRON CORP., WALTHAM, MASS.

T. A. Rosse
PRESIDENT
INSTRUMENTATION LABORATORY INC., WATERTOWN, MASS.

Francis J. Selvitelli
SENIOR DIGITAL APPLICATIONS ENGINEER
DYNAMICS RESEARCH CORP., WILMINGTON, MASS.

Meyer J. Shnitzler
CONSULTANT
THE GILLETTE COMPANY, BROOKLINE, MASS.

Lester Sodickson
SENIOR SCIENTIST
AMERICAN SCIENCE & ENGINEERING INC., CAMBRIDGE, MASS.

H. Sossen
EXECUTIVE VICE-PRESIDENT
HARVARD APPARATUS CO. INC., MILLIS, MASS.

R. Taylor
MEDICAL LIAISON ADMINISTRATOR
I.B.M., YORKTOWN HTS., N.Y.

Rhett Tsao
ADVISORY STATISTICIAN
I.B.M. CORPORATION, CAMBRIDGE, MASS.

A. Edward Urkiewicz
PRESIDENT
CARDIOVASCULAR INSTRUMENT CORP., WAKEFIELD, MASS.

William Zimmerman
PROJECT MANAGER, ADVANCED PROGRAMS DEPARTMENT
AVCO WILMINGTON RESEARCH CENTER, WILMINGTON, MASS.

M.I.T.–Harvard Participants

G. Octo Barnett
DIRECTOR OF THE LABORATORY OF COMPUTER SCIENCE
MASSACHUSETTS GENERAL HOSPITAL

H. Frederick Bowman
N.A.E. STUDY STAFF
MASSACHUSETTS INSTITUTE OF TECHNOLOGY

George B. Benedek
PROFESSOR OF PHYSICS
MASSACHUSETTS INSTITUTE OF TECHNOLOGY

Philip N. Bowditch
INSTRUMENTATION LABORATORY
MASSACHUSETTS INSTITUTE OF TECHNOLOGY

Gordon S. Brown
DEAN OF THE SCHOOL OF ENGINEERING
MASSACHUSETTS INSTITUTE OF TECHNOLOGY

Philip A. Drinker
CONSULTANT-SURGERY (ENGINEERING)
PETER BENT BRIGHAM HOSPITAL

Murray Eden
PROFESSOR OF ELECTRICAL ENGINEERING
MASSACHUSETTS INSTITUTE OF TECHNOLOGY

Joseph D. Fleming
INSTRUMENTATION LABORATORY
MASSACHUSETTS INSTITUTE OF TECHNOLOGY

Harriet L. Hardy
ASSISTANT MEDICAL DIRECTOR
MASSACHUSETTS INSTITUTE OF TECHNOLOGY

William B. Kannel
CLINICAL ASSOCIATE IN PREVENTIVE MEDICINE
HARVARD MEDICAL SCHOOL

Robert W. Mann
PROFESSOR OF MECHANICAL ENGINEERING
MASSACHUSETTS INSTITUTE OF TECHNOLOGY

William H. Matthews
N.A.E. STUDY STAFF
MASSACHUSETTS INSTITUTE OF TECHNOLOGY

Henry C. Meadow
ASSOCIATE DEAN
HARVARD MEDICAL SCHOOL

Edward W. Merrill
PROFESSOR OF CHEMICAL ENGINEERING
MASSACHUSETTS INSTITUTE OF TECHNOLOGY

Joseph F. O'Connor
ADMINISTRATIVE ASSISTANT TO VICE-PRESIDENT FOR SPECIAL LABORATORIES
MASSACHUSETTS INSTITUTE OF TECHNOLOGY

David M. Ozonoff
N.A.E. STUDY STAFF
MASSACHUSETTS INSTITUTE OF TECHNOLOGY

Barney Reiffen
LECTURER IN ELECTRICAL ENGINEERING
MASSACHUSETTS INSTITUTE OF TECHNOLOGY

John F. Rockart
ASSISTANT PROFESSOR OF MANAGEMENT
MASSACHUSETTS INSTITUTE OF TECHNOLOGY

Jack P. Ruina
VICE-PRESIDENT FOR SPECIAL LABORATORIES
MASSACHUSETTS INSTITUTE OF TECHNOLOGY

David D. Rutstein
RIDLEY WATTS PROFESSOR OF PREVENTIVE MEDICINE
HARVARD MEDICAL SCHOOL

Herbert Sherman
LEADER OF SPACE TECHNIQUES AND EQUIPMENT, LINCOLN LABORATORY
MASSACHUSETTS INSTITUTE OF TECHNOLOGY

Irwin W. Sizer
DEAN OF THE GRADUATE SCHOOL
MASSACHUSETTS INSTITUTE OF TECHNOLOGY

John B. Stanbury
PROFESSOR OF NUTRITION
MASSACHUSETTS INSTITUTE OF TECHNOLOGY

Louis D. Smullen
PROFESSOR OF ELECTRICAL ENGINEERING, HEAD OF THE DEPARTMENT
MASSACHUSETTS INSTITUTE OF TECHNOLOGY

Oleh J. Tretiak
LECTURER, ELECTRICAL ENGINEERING
MASSACHUSETTS INSTITUTE OF TECHNOLOGY

Laurence R. Young
ASSOCIATE PROFESSOR OF AERONAUTICS
MASSACHUSETTS INSTITUTE OF TECHNOLOGY

On September 12 and 13, 1968, a meeting was held at M.I.T. to discuss the potentials and problems of future university-industrial cooperation in the field of biomedical engineering. This meeting, conducted by the N.A.E. Study Steering Committee, was attended by approximately twenty-five faculty and staff members from M.I.T. and Harvard and over fifty representatives from thirty-one industrial corporations. The first day was devoted primarily to presentations to the industrial representatives, the second day to discussion and contributions by all the participants.

Gordon S. Brown, Dean of Engineering at M.I.T., welcomed the conferees on the morning of September 12. He discussed how the research in engineering and living systems and the coordination of this research have developed at M.I.T. and Harvard over the past several years. He outlined possibilities for future work in these areas and reviewed some of the general and administrative policies that would have to be established. Following these introductory remarks, Professor Murray Eden of M.I.T. explained the nature of the N.A.E. study. He described the approach taken by the two universities in establishing the task groups and in determining the areas of present and future concern.

Several of the Task Group chairmen presented the findings and recommendations of their committees. Dr. G. Octo Barnett discussed the report on medical care microsystems and described the development work in information processing that he is conducting at Massachusetts General Hospital. He outlined some of the specific problems in industrial-hospital relations resulting from the organizational structure of hospitals, which he characterized as "feudal systems." The strength of tradition in the medical community will make revolution impossible, he said, but we must look for ways to force evolutionary changes in the hospital power structure. He pointed out that present methods of hospital practice and operation are so archaic and inefficient that we cannot afford to perpetuate them, but that the forms of existing practices are so difficult to handle that no one has yet been able to really come to grips with them.

Professor John F. Rockart of M.I.T. then presented the program for research which was recommended by the regionalization of health services task group. Some

300

additional remarks on the possibilities of research in that area were given by Dr. Herbert Sherman of M.I.T.'s Lincoln Laboratory.

The next speaker was Professor Robert Mann, who had served as co-chairman of both the sensory aids and the skeletal prostheses and neuromuscular control task groups. After reviewing these reports, Professor Mann discussed the development of an artificial arm—the "Boston Arm"—whose initial research work had been done by M.I.T. graduate students. He explained that through the support and collaboration of Liberty Mutual Insurance Company, it had been possible for workers from M.I.T., the Massachusetts General Hospital, Harvard Medical School, and the company's rehabilitation division to evaluate this artificial arm and to develop it to an advanced prototype stage. He pointed out some of the advantages which accrued to both the universities and the company as a result of this joint effort.

The next speaker was Dr. Arthur Kantrowitz, vice-president of Avco Corporation and director of the Avco-Everett Research Laboratory. Dr. Kantrowitz defined two types of problems in biomedical engineering: those he termed "desiccated," i.e., totally specified, and therefore easily contained within conventional disciplinary boundaries, and which can be dealt with industrially on a pure profit basis; and those he considered as requiring collaboration in depth between biological investigators and engineers. With respect to support of research, Dr. Kantrowitz pointed out that the federal government has proved to be extremely powerful financially and that it must use that power in this emerging area, which is also relatively new to industry, if meaningful research efforts are to be mounted. He expressed pessimism about the prospects of obtaining substantial new support and suggested, therefore, that the engineering profession be better represented in the decision-making circles of government agencies concerned with the support of biomedical research—particularly research in those areas of investigation requiring creativity in engineering. He advocated balanced representation of engineers and biologists in all such policy-making bodies. The N.A.E. report ought to help define the structure of and build the new policy-making entity.

With respect to industrial research in biomedical engineering, Dr. Kantrowitz urged that industries be willing to perform government research on a contract basis and to publish and disclose all research results. He argued that the withholding of proprietary information would make it impossible to maintain first-class research over a period of years and suggested that the spin-off from research would justify corporate capital investment by private industry, provided that research expenses were fully borne by the government. This concept was discussed among the industrial representatives. It was clear that both sides of the argument were well represented.

The first speaker of the afternoon was Dr. Jack P. Ruina, Vice-President for Special Laboratories at M.I.T. Dr. Ruina pointed out the paradox of American medicine: that spectacular medical feats such as heart transplants are occurring in this country, while infant mortality and longevity statistics indicate that we are far behind many other nations in these vital areas. While he felt that there was a growing government commitment to contribute to better national health, he predicted that this would probably not take the form of a total commitment. Thus, new priorities and a new government role will change only through evolutionary rather than revolutionary means. Dr. Ruina felt that the forces of the biomedical community were very different from those in the military-industrial complex or those on Madison Avenue. One of the most significant problems is the gaps between the producer, the manufacturer, and the consumer. According to Dr. Ruina, effective research and development seems to require a close interaction among these. The very high marketing expense also inhibits industrial efforts in this area. Dr. Ruina felt that the N.I.H. is not now equipped to handle large academic or industrial work in biomedical engineering. With respect to industry's role in the future, he suggested that it would probably not be financially fruitful for small companies to venture into these new, unproven fields. However, if large industrial firms were aggressive, they might uncover new markets. It is probable that ultimate success will depend on the government's assuming the roles of both supporter and consumer in this area, just as it has done in the space effort.

The next task group report was given by Professor

Edward Merrill of M.I.T. who discussed artificial internal organs. On the subject of industrial entrepreneurship in the burgeoning field of biomedical engineering (with specific reference to artificial organs), Professor Merrill felt there were two major problems: a very small market potential and the legal liability for death of patients with artificial organs. With respect to new health devices, conference attendees differed sharply on the questions of liability, and it was clear that this is an area which requires further definition and study. The role that Professor Merrill envisioned for industry is that of a subcontractor to the government in cooperation with universities.

At the conclusion of these presentations, Dr. Philip A. Drinker, a member of the N.A.E. Study Steering Committee, outlined four major categories for general group discussion:
1. Intellectual structure of university-hospital-industrial collaboration;
2. Economics of industrial participation;
3. Proprietary rights; and
4. Regulatory standards.
For purposes of illustration, Dr. Drinker described the research and development stages of a specific project carried out by university personnel and students in the hospital environment.

The salient features emerging during the meeting are summarized as follows:

1. Intellectual Structure of University-Hospital-Industrial Collaboration

Discussion centered on the basic problems of professional interaction among members of universities, hospitals and the communities they serve, and industry. A broad spectrum of problems was addressed, ranging from how an individual in a university identifies a complementary collaborator at a hospital or in industry (the identification of whom is necessary for successful collaboration and implementation of the problem at hand), to the effective placement, without exploitation, of the university thesis student in a hospital environment or in industry.

A good deal of the discussion, especially on the first

day, was directed at the problems—or rather the anxieties—of industrial people in attempting to interact with the university community in general, and the medical school and hospitals in particular. The anxieties are genuine, and the theme was a recurring one throughout much of the first day.

Foremost among these concerns was the question of who would be subordinate, or assistant, to whom in a collaborative effort. It was generally agreed that research is not an egalitarian process and that the man who generates a problem is the leader of the investigation. Actually, the situation is not really different at the bioengineering interface than it is in either biology (or medicine) or engineering. Man, however, is reluctant to play a subordinate role to anyone he does not consider a professional peer. The solution to this problem now rests primarily with the individuals participating in joint ventures and will depend on the success of newer educational programs.

There seems to be a clear and genuine educational need for the doctor, or biologist, and the engineer (both academic and industrial), to work in each other's area at least long enough to become familiar with his counterpart's problems and methods. Thus, it is quite likely that the academician will increase his development efforts (perhaps including some pilot-plant types of operation) within the university and the hospital environment and that research will grow in industry. It also seems clear that workers within each classification must avoid the tendency to stake out inviolable areas to be guarded jealously.

The participants at the meeting seemed to be in general accord on having more collaboration in the areas of research and development. The hope was expressed that mechanisms could be set up whereby industrial workers would join students and faculty in the early stages of research and that university members would get out into the industrial area during the later stages of development and early production of a device or during conversion of a concept or system to the public domain. Of particular importance in the area of device development is the need for the engineer to live for a time in the world of the hospital and become familiar with the technical problems of the doctor.

304

The inventor or developer of a device usually wants to stay with it. He would like to have his students continue participating in various phases of its progress. Professor Mann (M.I.T.) felt that this need not be a problem as he related experiences in the development of the Boston Arm.

Two areas of interaction between university-hospital complexes and industry—information exchange and personnel exchange—were discussed at some length. It was proposed that a clearing house or a "yellow pages" system be established which would include the names and interests of individuals from the university, medical care, and industrial communities. It was pointed out by one industrial representative that the yellow pages system may reveal esoteric problems of little general or commercial interest. What is wanted and needed here, however, is a vehicle by which problems can be taken to and solved by industry in the most efficient manner. Thus, the clearing house must also serve an advisory function.

One industrial representative suggested the creation of an "Office of Biomedical Implementation" that would take problems defined by the university or medical professor and then distribute them for industrial consultation and bidding. The necessity for industry to work in hospitals was rather firmly established.

---

2. Economics of Industrial Participation

Problem areas discussed here related to funding, research, development, marketing, techniques, and production. The consensus of the group was that the bulk of the money for research and development in the medical area has to come from government sources. There was a general feeling that it would be desirable for the government to create an administrative capacity that would do for development in biology and medicine what N.I.H. has heretofore done for other research development programs. It would include in its mandate the solicitation and distribution of development funds. Two levels of activity were discussed: the device level (local) and the health care system level (national). A second general consensus was that if the government is to play a major role in supporting development activity, it must also undertake, or underwrite, the broad market surveys which would clearly indicate for industry the financial impact of health care devices and systems.

Dr. Saul Aronow, a physicist representing an industrial firm and Massachusetts General Hospital, identified several problem areas he has noted in his experience.

1. The matter of whether the initiating physician or the industrial concern should finance the development?

2. The physician doesn't always know what he really wants; as a result of his having attempted much of the development himself before contacting engineering collaborators, he frequently obtains solutions for the wrong problems.

3. The problems that concern the physician are often technically trivial and lack significant market potential.

4. The research workers often make unrealistic evaluations of the market for the device.

5. Project secrecy and professional rivalry exist everywhere.

6. Medical customers are both fickle and individualistic. (The electronic stethoscope is a fine example: Lockheed supported the development costs of $100,000, only to find that the total market amounted to four devices).

The industrial firms interested in development made it clear that they want to be part of the early formulation of problems and not receive only totally defined projects that are of no further interest to the university members. The reasons for this were both motivational and technical; the new problem has more intrinsic interest, but far more important, the developer can do his job better if he is thoroughly versed in all facets of the problem.

It was agreed that there are two general classes of development project. In the first are the instruments or devices requiring substantial technologic development because they so specialized that only a few will be required. Here, financing must be by direct contract or subsidy, with the government either paying the costs or guaranteeing the market. The other consists of devices that may have a very large potential market—for example, the types of equipment that can be sold in quantity to hospitals or practicing physicians. In this latter group it was agreed that the real problem in development is not the first 5, 10, or even 100 models, because governmental subsidy, as in the former category, could provide the necessary mechanism. The fundamental difficulty is the transition to general availability in the public domain. It is only this latter phase of the transition that can provide the incentive for industry to pick up the idea and move with it. It was generally agreed that if a viable development organization could be established, an essential function would be the whole problem of market surveys, including both exploration and creation of new markets, in this rapidly evolving industry.

3. Proprietary Rights

This is a serious problem area and one that has to be faced squarely if large-scale interaction is to be successful. There appeared to be a desire on the part of some of the industrial representatives for an agency to play a third- or fourth-party role in university-industrial relationships. Arthur D. Little has a group that acts as liaison between inventors and licensees. The group searches out and recommends appropriate industrial concerns. Licensed commercial applications could also be a source of funds to both the innovator and the licensee. The general sense of the participants was that mechanisms for licensing commercial production are essential. There was some feeling that this should be extended a step further to provide for patenting and for distribution of royalties to individuals within the organization carrying out the research and development. Another problem of joint collaboration on research projects, often those with outside sources of funding, is that of the many different and usually contradictory patent policies, which may apply to the same project or device. A uniform or compatible patent policy is obviously an early requirement.

4. Regulatory Standards

The problems of standards that encompass safety, efficacy, uniform practices, and the many aspects of legal responsibility were also discussed. General questions of the manufacturing standards practiced by industry as a whole were reviewed. In those sectors of industry in which standards are self-imposed, efforts are generally limited to simple quality control, although some consideration may be given to the safety of the device and its compatibility with related, but noncompetitive, products of other manufacturers. (As examples, consider the interchangeability of batteries, spark plugs, and so on in the automative industry.) In general, it must be admitted that as far as the safety and health of the public consumer are concerned, such self-imposed standards are rarely, if ever, adequate, and then only in the areas of high competition; in noncompetitive segments of industry, manufacturing standards have never evolved without the influence of some type of regulatory or advisory agency, such as the Food and Drug Administration or the Underwriters Laboratory.

Some shortcomings and inadequacies in the powers exercised by these latter bodies were discussed. It was generally agreed that serious and concerted efforts must be made through some type of agency (such as the university-medical-industrial collaborative unit discussed at the conference) to establish a regulatory body for the control of biomedical devices; otherwise this function will fall to the government by default. The question was raised, but not resolved, as to whether by taking on this function a private institution or agency would eliminate itself as a potential developer of the devices it was empowered to approve or reject. One possibility would be for this collaborative organization to serve in an advisory capacity to a regulatory agency yet to be established.

Conclusions

There was clear and general agreement among all the participants of this conference that enhanced communication and collaboration among workers in universities, the medical care community, and industry can offer great benefits not only to society as a whole but also to the collaborating institutions. It was generally agreed that if the greatest potential is to be attained, the gap between development and theory must be bridged. When an exciting idea or device is conceived by the scientist and made functional by the engineering technologist, it must be carried beyond the development of a simple prototype. Much more needs to be done: the market must be determined, the device must be produced, distributed, and made generally available to the public, and finally, it must be used effectively in the maintenance of health and the prevention and treatment of disease. Any gaps in this transition process will prevent society's effective exploitation of the original concept or device. The great variety of resources and talents that must be brought to bear on this broad constellation of problems can be achieved through appropriate combinations of the strengths of the university and the medical care and industrial communities.

Index

Bunker Hill Life Services program, 235

Cambridge, Massachusetts, 223, 224–228, 236–237, 238–239, *244*
Cambridge City Hospital, 7, 232, 239
Cammarn, M. R., 142
Cannon, Walter B., 21–23
Cardiology, 127
Cardiovascular disease, 179–180, 195–196
Cardiovascular functioning, 116–117, 209–210, 213, 214
Case-Western Reserve School of Medicine, 97–98
Caspersson, Torbjorn S. W., 288
Castleman, P. A., 151n
Cell culture, 172
  see also Organ and cell culture and storage
Cell storage, *see* Organ and cell culture and storage
Cellular biology, 96–97
Cellular physiology, 92
Center for Community Health and Medical Care, 60
Charlestown, Massachusetts, 233
Chain, Ernest, 42
CHART, 237
Chemistry, 92, 96–97
Children's Hospital, 6, 7, 226, 243
Clinics, *see* Health care systems; Hospitals
Collen, M. F., 151n
Colton, Clark K., 205
Community
  industry relations, 303–309
  university relations, 223, 303–309
Computers, *see* Data processing; Image processing
Computer science, 215
Conference on Interactions between the University, Industrial, and Medical Care Communities, 295–309
Continuing education, *see* Education, continuing
Coronary disease, *see* Cardiovascular disease
Crandon, L. R. G., 189
CRT, 145
Cybernetics, 24–25, 279

Data banks, *see* Data processing
Data processing, 19, 46, 69
  and bioengineering curriculum, 92

in continuing education, 105–106, 107
in diagnostic instrumentation, 117–119
in diagnostic processes, 124, 125, 127–128
in image processing, 135–137
in medical care microsystems, 140–148
at the Instrumentation Laboratory, 182–183
in physiological monitoring, 176–177, 185
and physiological systems analysis, 202–219 *passim*
in regional health services, 224–228, 230, 232–234, 237–239, *244*
and sensory aids, 247–267 *passim*
and skeletal prostheses, 274
and subcellular engineering, 286–287, 291
  see also Image processing
Development, 20, 43–51, 52
  see also Models and devices
Devey, Gilbert, *13*
Devices, *see* Models and devices
Diagnosis, 187–188
  in continuing education, 105–106, 128
  data processing in, 117–119, 124, 127–128, 146–147
  instrumentation in, 20, 112–122
  research (proposed) in, 114–118
  see also Physiological monitoring; Physiological systems analysis
  and physiological monitoring, 186–187
  and regional health services, 233, 234
  processes in, 123–133
  research (proposed), 125–129
  see also Interdisciplinary relationships; Organizational structuring
Directors of medical education, 107–108, 110
Dow Chemical Company, 80
Dravid, A. N., 206
Drinker, Philip A., 6, 12n
Drugs, 198

Ebert, Robert H., 9
Economics, 140, 231
EDCO, 237
Eden, Murray, 12, *13*
Education in bioengineering, 27–38, 52–53, 58

312

Massachusetts Institute of Technology, 47
Center for Advanced Engineering Study, 14, 106, 108–109, 110, 111
Center for Community Health and Medical Care, 60
Center for Sensory Aids Evaluation and Development, 246, 247, 248, 256–257
  see also M.I.T., Department of Mechanical Engineering
Committee on Biomedical Engineering, 6
Department of Aeronautics, 79
Department of Biology, 5, 8, 98
Department of Chemical Engineering, 88, 281
Department of Chemistry, 8
Department of Electrical Engineering, 88, 247
Department of Material Sciences, 281
Department of Mechanical Engineering
  and bioengineering curriculum, 88
  and sensory aids, 246–247, 259
  Sensory Aids Group, 254–258, 262–264, 277
  and skeletal prostheses, 271, 280–281
Department of Metallurgy, 271
Department of Nuclear Engineering, 205
Department of Nutrition and Food Science, 8, 98
Electronic Systems Laboratory, 8
Engineering Projects Laboratory, 8
Health Service, 67
Practicing Engineer Advanced Study Program, 106
Research Laboratory of Electronics, 5, 8
  Cognitive Information Processing Group, 248–253
  and diagnostic instrumentation, 121
  and physiological systems analysis, 196
  and sensory aids, 246, 247–248
Sloan School of Management, 8, 60, 228, 277
Summer Study on Engineering (1967), 233
Urban Systems Group, 244
  see also Harvard University-Massachusetts Institute of Tech-

nology; Instrumentation Laboratory; Joint Center for Urban Studies of M.I.T. and Harvard; Lincoln Laboratory; National Magnet Laboratory; Research Reactor
Massachusetts Mental Health Center, 7
Mathematics, 19, 20, 21
  and artificial internal organs, 83
  and continuing education, 16, 31–33, 40–41, 88, 90–91, 108
  and information systems, 52, 54
  and medical care improvement, 59
  and physiological monitoring, 183
  and physiological systems analysis, 194, 195, 198, 214, 215
  and research, 39–40
Matthews, William H., 12n
Mead, Jere, 180
Meadow, Henry C., 12n
Meakins, Jonathan, 188
Medical care systems, 11, 27, 46, 47, 55–70, 138–152
  costs, 55, 240–241
  data processing in, 140–148
  and diagnostic processes, 125–128
  financial aspects of, 59–60, 68, 70
  flow patterns in, 63–64
  information processing in, 139, 142, 145–146
  institutional resources in, 65–66
  models, 58–70
  problems, 61–65, 302
  research (proposed), 140–148
  see also Financial structure; Health care systems; Hospitals; Interdisciplinary relations; Organizational structuring
Medical Electronic News, 119
Medical records, 142–146, 184, 230
Medicine, 16, 19, 21
  and artificial internal organs, 76
  and bioengineering curriculum, 31–33
  curative, 56, 57
  and information, 52
  and interfaces, 20
  and medical care systems, 11, 16, 58
  and models and devices, 305
  and physiological systems analysis, 204
  preventive, 56, 57
  organization of research in, 41–42

Organizational structuring (*continued*)
in skeletal prostheses research, 273–274, 276–277
in subcellular engineering research, 286–289, 292–293
Organ transplantation, 157–158
Orthopedics, *see* Skeletal prostheses
Otolaryngology, 217, 218
Otoneurology, 217, 218
Ozonoff, David M., 12n

Palovcek, F. P., 231n
Pandicio, A., 6
Pappalardo, Neil, 184
Paramedical personnel, 67, 144–145, 242
Parrish, Joseph, 8
Pathology, 45, 92, 110, 143, 203
see also Psychopathology
Personnel, allocation of
in artificial internal organs research, 81–82
in continuing education research, 111
in medical care systems, 66–68
research in, 149
in physiological systems analysis research, 202
in skeletal prostheses research, 272–274, 277, 278
Peter Bent Brigham Hospital, 5, 7, 177, 195
Peterson, Osler L., 6
Pharmocology, 92, 96–97, 101–102, 215–216
Photofluorometry, 98
Photometry, 98
see also Image processing
Physical sciences, 16, 19, 22, 39–40, 52, 59
Physicians, 29–30, 36–38, 109–110, 113–114, 120
see also Health care; Hospitals; Medical care systems
Physics, 21, 32–33, 90, 91
Physiological monitoring, 166–191
in biological control systems, 98, 100–102
data processing in, 176–177, 185
definition of, 173
and diagnosis, 186–187
and physiologic measurement, 19–20, 173–175, 189
problems in, 175–177, 178, 180
research (current), 174–176, 187–188

research (proposed), 172–173, 176–178, 180, 184–185, 186–187
see also Financial structuring; Interdisciplinary relationships; Organizational structuring
see also Biological control systems; Diagnosis, instrumentation in; Physiological systems analysis
Physiological systems analysis, 192–221
and biological control systems, 98, 100–102
continuing education in, 204–205
data processing in, 202–219 *passim*
research (current), 205–219
research (proposed), 195–198
see also Interdisciplinary relationships; Organizational structuring; Biological control systems; Diagnosis, instrumentation in; Physiological monitoring; Physiology
Physiologic measurement, *see* Physiological monitoring
Physiology, 3, 20–21, 39, 45, 56
and bioengineering curriculum, 90
and biological control systems, 95–96, 99–102
and continuing education, 110
and homeostasis, 21, 23, 25–26
kidney, 6
and subcellular engineering, 291
and telemetry, 100–102
Poitras, Jim, 184
Postural control, 203
Professional Activities Study, 142
Programmed learning, 105
Programmed teaching, 34
Psychopathology, 211
see also Pathology
Psychotherapy, 211
Public health, *see* Health care systems
Public law, 89–239, 61
Pulmonary functioning, 116
Pusey, Nathan M., 9

Record processing, 118
Reid, R. C., 206
Research, 20–21, 27, 39–42, 50, 52, 56
see also Development; Financial structure; Organizational structuring; Personnel
Research Reactor, 8

318

Weinman, I., 28
Weiss, Soma, 187, 188
West Roxbury Veterans Hospital,
    7
Whipple, George C., 4
Wiener, Norbert, 24
Wiesner, Jerome, 9
Wilmington, Delaware, 237
Wolff, H., 187, 191n

"Yellow pages" system, *see* Information systems
Young, L. R., 6

Zachary, Norman, 6